Diabetes

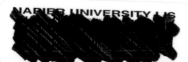

A Tavistock Professional Book

The Experience of Illness

Series Editors: Ray Fitzpatrick and Stanton Newman

Diabetes

David Kelleher

Routledge

First published in 1988 by
Routledge
11 New Fetter Lane, London EC4P 4EE

© 1988 David Kelleher

Phototypeset in 10/12 pt Linotron Times by Input Typesetting Ltd,
London

Printed in Great Britain by Richard Clay Ltd, Bungay, Suffolk

British Library Cataloguing in Publication Data
Kelleher, David, *1935–*
    Diabetes.
    1. Man. Diabetes
    I. Title   II. Series
    616.4'62

    ISBN 0–415–00725–9 Hbk
    ISBN 0–415–00726–7 Pbk

Contents

Editors' preface

Diabetes particularly illustrates the dilemma arising out of the success of modern health care. Treatments such as insulin have rightly been hailed as major breakthroughs in twentieth-century medicine. For many sufferers of diabetes the chances of good health and a satisfying quality of life are now realistic possibilities. Yet, as understanding of the dietary and other behavioural influences upon the course of diabetes increases, treatment imposes further demands on the individual.

David Kelleher explores the lives of a group of diabetics. He draws on their accounts of their experiences of the disorder and illustrates the force of social background in structuring the reality of the disorder, by letting the sufferers speak for themselves. Many of the samples he draws on in this volume are in manual occupations, and they graphically reveal the conflicts between work, other social pressures, and the demands of treatment regimens. A central theme running through this volume is the problematic concept of control. On the one hand the therapeutic objective is to control blood sugar levels; on the other hand adherence to the many demands of treatment may be experienced as control over one's life. He also draws attention to the important current debates about the goals and objectives of health care for individuals with diabetes and about the most appropriate forms of providing care.

This book is one of a series of volumes which attempts to bring together the accumulating sociological and psychological research on major contemporary health problems. This body of thought is increasingly seen as essential in the education and practice of health professionals.

Chapter one

Diabetes mellitus, its nature and prevalence

Introduction

Diabetes is a chronic, incurable disease whose treatment imposes severe constraints on the lives of sufferers. Although it has been recognized for at least 3,000 years it is still imperfectly understood. The treatment of diabetes and the life chances of diabetics have been much improved since the discovery of insulin in 1922, but it is a difficult disorder to manage and much of the responsibility for the day-to-day management lies with the diabetic person. This chapter discusses evidence and debates about the nature of the disease, its variability, and distribution in the world.

The nature of diabetes

The raised level of blood glucose is the central feature of diabetes, although it is just one sign in a complex of metabolic processes. The raised glucose level is itself caused by the failure of the pancreas to produce insulin or the failure of the receptor cells in the tissues of the body to be able to utilize the insulin which is produced. Insulin plays a crucial part in conjunction with glucagon in controlling the level of glucose in the blood and it is also important in the process by which the body's cells take up glucose and use it as energy. The inability to use insulin leads to high concentrations of fatty acids and glycerol, and to ketones developing in the urine, thus bringing about a loss of protein which reduces the body's ability to grow new tissue and repair damaged tissue. The body's immune defence system against bacterial and fungal invasion is also reduced.

Although the basis of any definition of diabetes mellitus is the existence of a raised level of blood glucose (hyperglycaemia), diabetes is no longer thought of as a single disease entity. It appears to have several different aetiologies, presents in a number of ways, may progress to a variety of different pathological consequences, and involves various treatments.

Types of diabetes

Several different principles have been used to classify the variety of diabetic phenomena. This book will follow the WHO report (1985: 18) which recommends that three major clinical sub-classes of diabetes should be recognized:

1 insulin-dependent diabetes mellitus (IDDM)
2 non-insulin-dependent diabetes mellitus (NIDDM)
  (a) non-obese
  (b) obese
3 malnutrition-related diabetes mellitus (MRDM)

Several other less common types of diabetes 'associated with certain conditions and syndromes' are also recognized: (1) pancreatic disease, (2) disease of hormonal aetiology, (3) drug-induced or chemical-induced conditions, (4) abnormalities of insulin or its receptors, (5) certain genetic syndromes, and (6) miscellaneous. There is also a category of 'impaired glucose tolerance' where the level is above normal but below that recognized as diabetes and a further category of gestational diabetes for those just diagnosed during pregnancy.

Insulin-dependent diabetes (IDDM)

The great majority of cases of diabetes which occur in children are of the insulin-dependent type which was why the category of 'juvenile-onset' was previously used. 'Type I' has also been used as the name for this type of diabetes. Typically the onset of the classical symptoms of greatly increased thirst, polyuria, wasting, and ultimately coma is sudden. Population studies have indicated a peak incidence occurring around the age of 10 to 13 years with the highest rates occurring in Caucasian populations. The presenting symptoms when supported by evidence of greatly elevated concentrations of glucose and ketones in the blood and urine lead to the diagnosis of insulin-dependent diabetes and insulin treatment is prescribed.

Non-insulin-dependent diabetes (NIDDM)

About 80 per cent of diabetics have this form of diabetes. It is usually diagnosed in middle age and the prevalence increases with age. It may, however, occur at a younger age, particularly in some populations (Pima Indians in the USA for example). The symptoms of increased thirst, polyuria, tiredness, and skin irritations may be accompanied by obesity and often appear insidiously over a period of time with hyperglycaemia having been present for several years before diagnosis. Some cases of non-insulin-dependent diabetes later need insulin treatment. This is sometimes the result of failing to comply with the treatment required but the WHO report (1985: 26) suggests that 'in most cases it probably represents the progressive natural history of NIDDM'. A substantial proportion of NIDDM people are not obese and the WHO report therefore recommends that the two classes of NIDDM, obese and non-obese, be recognized. Non-insulin-dependent diabetics were formerly known as 'maturity-onset' or Type II diabetics, or, in the case of young people, as maturity-onset diabetes of the young (MODY).

Malnutrition-related diabetes (MRDM)

Evidence from tropical developing countries has shown that young diabetics, adults, and children, often present with a pattern of symptoms different from those recognized in populations of developed countries. The young patients may be grossly underweight and have other signs of malnutrition. It is suggested that there are two sub-classes of MRDM, fibrocalculous pancreatic diabetes and protein-deficient pancreatic diabetes. The WHO report (1985: 21 and 23) states that the key metabolic features are:

> moderate to severe hyperglycaemia that requires insulin for control, sometimes in high doses, and the absence of ketosis (pancreatic diabetes)

3

or

resistance to the development of ketosis, partial resistance to the action of insulin, extreme degrees of wasting (protein deficient type).

Symptoms

In the case of young people the presenting symptoms of diabetes are directly caused by the deficiency of insulin and the high level of blood glucose. The symptoms are usually a severe thirst and an increased volume of urine; these may be accompanied by loss of weight and drowsiness or even a state of coma.

Older people may also present with these symptoms but in most cases their symptoms are less clear cut. Their problems may stem from a reduction in the amount of insulin they are able to produce, but may also be the result of a gradually developed inability to make use of the insulin they produce. The presenting symptoms may include feeling thirsty, feeling tired, and skin irritations particularly around the genital areas. In some cases they may be overweight. Keen (1983) noted that there may be no symptoms at the time of diagnosis in the case of middle-aged diabetics as the diagnosis may be made in the course of a routine blood or urine test.

The long-term effect of diabetes

Both non-insulin-dependent diabetics and insulin-dependent diabetics run the risk of developing 'complications' of diabetes, which include retinopathy (damage to the retina) leading to impaired vision and in some cases blindness; nephropathy (damage to the kidney) which can cause kidney failure; neuropathy (damage to the nerve fibres of either the peripheral nerves or the autonomic nervous system). Damage to the peripheral nerves often affects the legs and feet of diabetics making them less aware of pain and sensation and more susceptible to infection and in some cases gangrene. Damage to the autonomic nervous system may affect bladder control and blood pressure and may cause impotence.

Retinopathy is now recognized as the commonest cause of blindness in the UK. Prevalence studies of eye damage resulting from diabetes (retinopathy) show variations according to the age at diagnosis and the duration of diabetes. Those diagnosed as diabetic after the age of 50 may already be suffering from retinopathy at the time of diagnosis. Diabetes may affect the eyes of both insulin-dependent and non-insulin-dependent diabetics. A study conducted in the USA showed that for those diagnosed as diabetic before the age of 30, the prevalence of retinopathy varies from 17 per cent for those who had had diabetes for less than five years to as much as 97.5 per cent for those who had had diabetes for more than fifteen years (Jarrett 1986: 51). Severe retinopathy is less common and the rate varies from 6.6 per cent in London to 12.3 per cent in Tokyo (Keen and Ekoe 1984). Blindness has been found to develop in about one-third of young-onset insulin-dependent diabetics after about forty years and in about 10 per cent of non-insulin-dependent diabetics (WHO 1985). However it must be stressed that early recognition of retinopathy can lead to treatment which limits the damage.

About 50 per cent of insulin-dependent diabetics are likely to develop kidney disease (nephropathy) and about 4–5 per cent will develop a severe form. This will necessitate dialysis or a renal transplant for some (National Kidney Research Fund Report 1987). Non-insulin-dependent diabetics may also develop nephropathy but there are wide geographic variations in the prevalence rates.

Diabetic neuropathy causes chronic foot problems in about 5 per cent of diabetics and the incidence of gangrene amongst diabetics is 0.5 per cent (WHO 1985). The prevalence of neuropathy in diabetic patients with good long-term glycaemic control is approximately 10 per cent but in patients with poor long-term glycaemic control two-thirds can be expected to develop clinical neuropathy within twenty-five years (Clements 1986).

The main concern in the treatment of diabetics is to reduce blood glucose levels to near normal in order to eliminate or reduce the symptoms and to reduce the risk of developing the long-term complications. The WHO report (1985) describes the range aimed at in treatment procedures:

The range of glucose concentrations aimed for in treatment is similar to normal and falls within the following limits: 3.3–5.6

mmol glucose/litre (60–100 mg/dl) of venous whole blood under fasting conditions and not exceeding 10 mmol/litre (180 mg/dl) after meals; blood glucose concentration should not be allowed to fall below 3 mmol/litre (55 mg/dl).

The evidence that close control of blood glucose levels will prevent the development of complications is not conclusive but most authorities agree that complications are more likely to appear when the metabolic control of diabetes, the control of blood glucose levels, is poor. Greene (1986), reporting on a long-term prospective study of 4,400 non-insulin-dependent diabetics, states that the complications of nephropathy, neuropathy, and retinopathy increased with the duration of diabetes and that all three were more common in diabetic patients in whom metabolic control was poor.

Apart from the risk of experiencing diabetic complications and a premature death from diabetes, diabetics also have a two to three times higher risk of dying from coronary heart disease compared with non-diabetics. This risk is greatest in industrialized countries and is a greater comparative risk for women than for men. In developing countries there is an increased risk of stroke resulting from diabetes-related hypertension.

In industrialized countries the life expectancy of early-onset IDDM is approximately three-quarters that of non-diabetics and in the case of non-insulin-dependent diabetics life expectancy is reduced by several years. As a cause of death diabetes ranks high in many industrialized countries although its role as an underlying cause of death is often understated (Fuller 1983; Hamman 1983). In the USA more deaths are caused by diabetes than by lung cancer, breast cancer, motor accidents, or infant mortality. The USA mortality figure for 1979 was 14.8 per 100,000 for all age groups but 148.5 per 100,000 for the over-75 age group (WHO 1985).

Differences in incidence and prevalence

A striking feature of diabetes is the considerable extent to which it varies from one population to another. The highest incidence rates of IDDM have been found to be in developed countries such as Finland (Jarrett 1986: 13) but some of the highest incidence rates of NIDDM have been found in developing countries, in particular in the Pacific island of Nauru where the prevalence is thought to be around 30 per cent in the adult population (Zimmet 1982; Bennett 1983; WHO 1985). Other populations reported as having high prevalence of NIDDM are Mexican Americans (17 per cent), Israel (15.9 per cent), Fiji (13.5 per cent), (WHO 1985). High prevalence rates have also been reported amongst Indians living in Cape Town, South Africa (Bennett 1983), yet other ethnic groups living in the same city have much lower rates. There are clearly enormous difficulties in making sense of such variations in pattern, even when only developed, industrialized countries are compared (Hamman 1983). For the period 1976–8 Belgium had the high rate of 13.9 per 100,000 male deaths recorded as due to diabetes, whereas the nearby countries of Holland (Netherlands) and Britain had much lower rates (both 5.8 per 100,000 male deaths).

One serious problem in interpreting these differences is the variety of methods used to ascertain and interpret blood sugar levels (Keen and Ekoe 1984) and because there may be many undiagnosed cases in some populations (WHO 1985: 28). The British Diabetic Association for example estimates that there are probably as many as 600,000 undiagnosed diabetics in Britain. A further difficulty is establishing the threshold of glucose into- lerance at which diabetes is diagnosed. There are some who show signs of glucose intolerance but not at a high enough level to be classified as diabetic. About two-thirds of people in this category may go on to become diabetic and about one-third of them return to normal glucose tolerance. They pose particular problems when considering incidence in different populations. Indeed some commentators stress the arbitrary nature of the current classification:

The degrees of hyperglycaemia which qualify for the diagnosis of diabetes mellitus are now based upon the findings in large normal population samples and validated by prospective observations on outcome. However, they remain to some extent arbitrary lines drawn across 'a continuous distribution' of values in most populations.

(Keen 1983: 168)

One attempt to achieve uniformity across countries is that of the

World Health Organisation which recommends diagnostic criteria both for clinical use in relation to individuals and for use in epidemiological studies. It suggests that when symptoms are present a single blood glucose estimation in excess of 11.1 mmol/litre (capillary, whole blood) establishes the diagnosis. This procedure may be sufficient even when symptoms are slight or absent, but where the blood glucose values do not establish the diagnosis for certain (that is they may lie just outside the certainty level) an oral glucose tolerance test (OGTT) is recommended. This involves measuring the blood glucose values after fasting and two hours after being given a drink of 75 g of glucose in 250–300 ml of water. In the case of children the test load of glucose should be related to their body weight. In the case of epidemiological studies attempting to assess the prevalence of glucose intolerance and diabetes the blood glucose concentration can be measured by the oral glucose tolerance test (WHO 1985).

Despite the difficulties of assessment the variation that has been identified is one potentially exciting way in which the causes of diabetes may be explored. Some evidence suggests that high prevalence rates may be associated with the relative affluence and sedentary life-styles commonly found in industrialized societies. For example rates of 5–10 per cent are reported in Sweden and the USA. In other industrialized countries rates are somewhat lower, for example Britain has rates of 2–5 per cent, while in Japan prevalence rates are 3 per cent. In contrast certain non-industrialized communities report rates of less than 1 per cent. The populations with the lowest rates are reported as being Eskimos and Alaskan Athabascan Indians (Zimmet 1982; Bennett 1983).

One hypothesis that may account for the above findings is that the level of over-eating and obesity and the sedentary life-style commonly found in developed, industrial societies are implicated in causing non-insulin-dependent diabetes. Such a hypothesis finds dramatic support in one case of rapid economic development. The Naurans, the inhabitants of a small island in the Pacific, have recently developed a prevalence rate of NIDDM of epidemic proportions at the same time as they have become more affluent, abandoned their traditional diet, and imported more of their food from Australia. They have also reduced the amount of manual work they perform and adopted a more sedentary life-style. In an epidemiological overview of NIDDM prevalence Zimmet (1982) provides more general support for the view that a community changing to a 'westernized' life-style is likely to experience an increase in the prevalence of non-insulin-dependent diabetes.

There are problems, however, with the simple explanation of diabetes as a 'disease of affluence' (Keen *et al.* 1978). There are difficulties in dietary surveys in isolating the part played by any one item of diet such as fat or sugar in causing diabetes. Nutritional factors may be important in both the causation of diabetes and its development but the adiposity often associated with NIDDM is not simply a result of over-eating. There is a further problem with the suggestion that diabetes is likely to become more prevalent with the spread of urban living and sedentary life-styles (Bennett 1983). The increased longevity of people in developed countries contributes to the relatively higher prevalence of NIDDM in these societies. Lipson (1986) estimates that 10 per cent of Americans aged 60 and 16–20 per cent of those aged 80 are diabetic. The higher incidence of diabetes in these societies may therefore be primarily a by-product of increased lifespan.

Evidence of the role of environmental factors may be obtained from the distribution of diabetes within societies. Whereas IDDM is more prevalent in social classes I and II, NIDDM is more prevalent in social classes IV and V in England and Wales (Hamman 1983). The link between social class and the risk of developing diabetes was examined in a study by Barker, Gardner, and Power (1982), when nine British towns were rated as having good or bad economic and social conditions on the basis of the income levels of residents, the percentage of car-owners, unemployment levels, and overcrowding in housing. There seemed to be no link between the incidence of IDDM and the economic and social conditions, but the incidence of NIDDM was considerably higher in the poorer towns. This pattern is supported by North American data that also link a high prevalence of diabetes with low social class (*Lancet* 1982). One contributing factor may be that obesity is more common amongst families with a low income.

When considering the varying incidence of diabetes in different social groups another hypothesis emerges. For example in the case of Fiji there are two main ethnic groups, with genetic differences between the groups. The Melanesian group had low prevalence rates among both the urban dwellers and those living in rural areas. The other group are Indians and both the urban dwellers and those living in rural surroundings had high prevalence rates. The rural Indians are subsistence farmers who are not obese, are physically active, and have a relatively poor diet. Their high prevalence rate seems likely therefore to be strongly influenced by a genetic susceptibility. Genetic influences may constitute an alternative hypothesis to that of environmental differences.

Studies of migrants may be particularly useful in teasing out the relative contributions of genetic and environmental factors in the causes of ill health. If the prevalence of diabetes in a migrant group alters to become similar to that of the host country it would suggest the importance of factors in the shared environment. If the prevalence rates of the migrant group continue to resemble those of the country of origin, genetic factors would seem to be important. Studies of migrant Indians illustrate some of the problems and possibilities of this kind of work in diabetes. The evidence from a range of studies indicates that in developed countries migrant Indians tend to have a higher prevalence of diabetes than others in the host country. This is consistent with a genetic interpretation. However, migrant Indians also have a higher prevalence rate than Indians who remain behind in India. The migrants are often economically in a better position than those who remain in India and so it seems that factors such as increased wealth produce changes in life-style which interact with their genetic susceptibility (Taylor and Zimmet 1983). In practice, in such examples, it is not clear how typical of an ethnic group migrants are and how much of their traditional culture and eating habits they retain in their new environment (Taylor and Zimmet 1983).

Evidence from studying identical twins, who have the same genetic make-up, suggests that there is a greater likelihood of non-insulin-dependent diabetes being affected by genetic inheritance than is the case for insulin-dependent diabetes. In a study of fifty-three pairs of identical twins, in forty-eight cases both twins were found to be non-insulin-dependent diabetics, giving a concordance rate of 90 per cent (Leslie and Pyke 1985: 58). In the case of insulin-dependent diabetes, where one twin is IDDM in 50 per cent of cases the other twin is also an insulin-dependent diabetic, that is the concordance rate is 50 per cent (Spencer and Cudworth 1983: 109).

One can also study other familial relations for evidence of genetic factors. A study of NIDDM conducted in India reported that in a sample of families in which both parents were NIDDM, 55.6 per cent of their children aged 40 or over also had non-insulin-dependent (as in Mohan, Ramachandran, and Viswanathan 1985). Such studies also provide further supporting evidence for the view that IDDM and NIDDM are two distinct types of diabetes as the relatives of people with IDDM are no more likely to develop NIDDM than are people with no diabetes in their genetic background (Leslie and Pyke 1985: 58).

An alternative method of investigating genetic factors is to seek evidence of specific biological markers. Research into genetic markers for diabetes suggest that susceptibility to IDDM may be conferred by genes of the HLA-DR4 allele being strongly associated with IDDM in all ethnic groups, and the HLA-DR3 allele showing an IDDM association only in Caucasian and some black populations. NIDDM is not HLA associated and as yet no specific marker of NIDDM has been identified (WHO 1985).

Genetic factors are implicated in both insulin-dependent and non-insulin-dependent diabetes, but in neither case is the genetic pattern a straightforward one (Keen 1987). It seems likely that other factors besides genetic ones are necessarily involved in both cases. For this reason, bodies such as the WHO are very reluctant to advocate policies of prevention of diabetes through genetic counselling and certainly do not discourage diabetics from having children.

Intervention

Investigation into the causes of diabetes is ultimately concerned with ways in which the disease may be prevented or ameliorated, most obviously by altering the environment. Environmental intervention would be clearly most effective with the recently defined third type of diabetes, malnutrition-related diabetes (MRDM). In the case of one sub-type of MRDM, protein-deficient pancreatic diabetes (PDPD) which is common in countries such as Bangladesh, Ghana, and Jamaica, the link is with a diet deficient in proteins leading to the development of diabetes.

In the case of IDDM and NIDDM the potential for environmental manipulation is less clear. Besides the general notions of an affluent life-style, more specific environmental factors have been suggested with specific populations. One study considered a particular dietary factor; Helgason and Jonasson (1981) suggested a direct link between an item of diet and the development of IDDM. They suggest that the seasonal peak in the incidence of diabetes in October-born children in Iceland could be explained by the presence of a recently developed preservative agent, nitrosamines, used in the curing of mutton which is traditionally eaten by Icelanders in the fortnight after Christmas. The role of nitrosamines perhaps needs to be examined further but is unlikely to explain more than a small part of the increase in prevalence associated with changes in diet.

A very different line of enquiry has been followed by Spencer and Cudworth (1983) who consider the evidence relating viral infections to the development of insulin-dependent diabetes. Studies have shown the Coxsackie B4 virus to be implicated in some cases; others have reported that diabetes has developed after patients have had mumps. Hamman (1983) reports on a Scottish study which appears to link overcrowding in housing and areas with a high population density with the risk of developing diabetes after viral infections. The reported seasonal peaks in the incidence of diabetes (Durranty, Ruiz, and Garcia de la Rios 1979) also lends some support to the belief that viral infections may be involved as the peaks do seem to coincide with periods when viral infections are common, but Spencer and Cudworth come to the conclusion that at present there is no clear evidence linking any one virus or group of virus with beta cell damage and the onset of IDDM.

Prevention of insulin-dependent diabetes is not possible in the present state of knowledge. The evidence concerning the part played by environmental factors in the causation of non-insulin-dependent diabetes does give some grounds for thinking that preventive action could be taken in selected communities. The WHO report (1985) discusses this possibility, suggesting that physical inactivity, a high fat diet, and obesity could be the most important risk factors to be tackled, at the same time emphasizing the need for further research to confirm that these are the most important factors. Certainly diabetes is a growing health problem and the costs to individuals and to society are considerable; it is important that attention should be given to seeking methods of prevention and improving the existing treatments.

The roles of genetic and environmental factors are not mutually exclusive and any explanation for diabetes will have to be mutifactorial. In addition diabetes appears to be made up of a family of disorders where the causal explanations might well differ.

Treatment

There are three basic aspects of treatment: insulin injections, diet, and tablets. Insulin-dependent diabetics are treated with daily, or more usually twice daily, injections of insulin. In most cases the insulin injections are administered by the patients themselves about 15–20 minutes before eating. The insulin, which is injected subcutaneously, is then dispersed via the bloodstream to assist the cells of the body tissues in the process of utilizing the food. There are three basic types of insulin used, the difference between them being mainly in the length of time they remain active in the body. Rapid-acting insulin starts to work soon after being injected but does not remain active for long; a second type has zinc added to it to slow down the rate at which it is used and so it remains active for a longer period; a third type also has zinc added to it and remains active for a long period. Some diabetics have been fitted with a pump attached to the stomach which supplies them with a continuous supply of insulin but the pump has to be refilled approximately every three days.

Insulin-dependent diabetics are also required to control their food intake. The dietary recommendations for IDDM diabetics were revised in 1983 by the British Diabetic Association and less emphasis is now placed on the diet being low in carbohydrates; more emphasis is placed on reducing fat intake, increasing the fibre content, and on balancing the overall energy content with insulin dosage and energy expenditure. Diabetics are expected to achieve this balance by knowing the calorific values of food eaten and by testing their blood sugar levels to see whether they are high or low. Urine samples may be tested instead of blood but the level of glucose in the urine is not always close to that in the blood and it is therefore a less accurate check on the level of blood glucose and the amount of insulin required. The treatment of IDDM diabetics is therefore aimed at achieving a blood glucose level which is near to that of non-diabetics. This requires careful attention, on a daily basis, to food intake, physical activity level, and insulin requirement.

Non-insulin-dependent diabetics may be treated by diet alone or by diet and tablets. Those controlled by diet alone are usually required to eat meals which are low in refined carbohydrates and fat. Alcohol consumption should also be restricted. The aim of the diet is usually to reduce weight and prevent obesity so that the insulin which is produced naturally is able to utilize the food as energy.

About 20–40 per cent of non-insulin-dependent diabetics need oral hypoglycaemic tablets as well as a dietary regimen to control their diabetes. These are of two main types, suphonylureas and biguanides. The sulphonylureas act to stimulate the production of insulin in the pancreas while the major effect of biguanides is to increase the effective take-up of glucose by the body tissues. Non-insulin-dependent diabetics taking oral hypoglycaemic tablets are also required to restrict their food intake and avoid obesity. Physical activity is encouraged in all diabetics and food used as energy is a part of the equation which equals good metabolic control.

There has been uncertainty as to whether 'complications' can be prevented by strict adherence to glycaemic control; there is widespread faith that good metabolic control will prevent the development of complications. However, Siperstein *et al.* came to the conclusion that studies attempting to show that good control of blood glucose prevented complications were, 'at best, inconclusive' (1977: 1,060). Other reviews came to similar conclusions. More recently, however, the balance of opinion has become much more optimistic about the effects of metabolic control (West 1982).

Particular issues remain to be resolved, for example whether the critical factor in the development of complications is the duration of the metabolic disorder or the degree of disturbance is still unclear. Nevertheless metabolic control remains at the heart of the medical management of diabetes.

Chapter two

The experience of diabetes

Diabetes is a disorder of metabolism, the effects of which may be so numerous and varied that delineation of typical experiences will inevitably prove difficult. The disorder may be well controlled and barely impinge on the sufferer's well-being or may substantially affect health. This chapter describes some of the central symptoms, problems, and patterns of the disorder, as experienced and reported by diabetics themselves.

Initial symptoms and diagnosis

Insulin-dependent diabetics most often develop symptoms in childhood, frequently around the age of puberty. Typically they experience symptoms of weight loss, drowsiness, excessive thirst and excessive urination. In some cases these symptoms may have developed into a loss of consciousness, a diabetic coma. There is sometimes a significant period of time between the onset of symptoms and diagnosis. A woman of 23 described the extensive range of symptoms she experienced before she was diagnosed at the age of 12:

> I lost weight, drinking, passing a lot of water and just literally passing out . . . me Dad used to carry me over to the GP and he put it down to periods for two months. In the end I couldn't even go to school 'cause in the classrooms I was running out every few minutes for a drink . . . I used to spend me dinner money on bottles of lemonade.

Another insulin-dependent woman described her symptoms immediately before she was diagnosed when pregnant:

> I'd take six glasses of water, line them up beside the bed,
> drink them, run off to the loo, fill them up again on the way
> back and that was how I spent the night.

Her diabetes was discovered when she went for a hospital ante-
natal check-up.

Some non-insulin-dependent diabetics may have symptoms that
take the individual to the doctor, for example weight increase,
feelings of tiredness, skin infections from cuts which have been
slow to heal, or a succession of eye or other infections. By
contrast, many others are quite often asymptomatic and diagnosed
in the course of other medical check-ups or eye tests. The main
sign is likely to be a raised blood sugar level. This may have
already caused damage to the eyes and the diabetes may become
apparent only in an examination of the eyes.

For those without symptoms, the diagnosis is, of course, quite
unexpected. One woman who had no symptoms describes how
she was alerted to her diabetes when she went for a job in the
catering industry:

> I went for an employment interview . . . the lady there said I
> should see my doctor when I got home.

For others mild or unnoticed symptoms are only related to
diabetes after diagnosis. As one diabetic explained:

> I used to feel thirsty but that I used to put down to the weather
> or hard work or something like that. But now I realize it
> could have been diabetes.

His thirst became more excessive and a relative who was a doctor
then advised him to see his GP.

The initial reaction to being told the diagnosis for many is
surprise or shock. This may be the case even though they have
presented with symptoms.

> I didn't believe it. Even now I think someone is going to be
> able to come along and tell me why my pancreas isn't
> working. They'll give me a tablet and it'll start again.

Others are frightened:

> It was just a shock to me. . . . I'm still a bit frightened because
> I don't feel well.

Diagnosis may bring people relief as for the first time they have an explanation for worrying symptoms. A medical diagnosis may also provide a more acceptable interpretation of symptoms. One man explained that his wife had mistaken his tiredness for laziness:

It was a good thing really that they did find out. It was starting to cause a bit of animosity, with the tiredness affecting. . . . It wasn't very nice. You'd come home from work and the next minute you were away [asleep] and the missus getting very upset . . . but once she found out, it sort of helped things, you know.

One factor that can influence immediate responses to diagnosis is prior knowledge of the disorder. Some people know what is involved when they are diagnosed diabetic because they have relatives who have experienced the disorder. Others know very little about diabetes and are unaware of the dangers of long-term complications. One woman felt no particular reaction when she was diagnosed:

Well, I didn't have any feelings actually, because I didn't know nothing about it, because there was nobody in the family that's got it.

Adjusting to treatment

Once diagnosed, the diabetic has immediately to come to terms with the many complex requirements of monitoring and treatment, which may be as demanding as any symptoms. Thus some patients may have immediately to learn a number of different new skills with regard to carrying out injections, monitoring their needs for injections, and achieving precise dosages. All of these may create new concerns. For example a newly diagnosed diabetic expressed his main worry:

Measuring the actual needle capsule, that worried me, on measurement. I may just accidentally put too much or too little in. I'm going to really have to pay attention to that.

For most diabetics the normally pleasurable and taken-for-granted activity of eating becomes something to be planned and evaluated. Thus for some being diagnosed diabetic results in a changed view of food. It can no longer be seen as one of the pleasures of life to be indulged in, but as something that has to be controlled, and eating comes to be surrounded by conflicting emotions. One newly diagnosed diabetic recounted the struggle he had to resist buying a Danish pastry in a self-service restaurant:

> I went down to have lunch in Regent Street and I was walking along and I picked out a roll with a certain level of carbohydrate, and I walked along to the cash desk, passing the Danish pastries. As I went to pay, it was a case of, I can't resist it [Danish pastry] and I ran back, quite true, and I ran back . . . I just couldn't resist it. I stopped and I thought, you mustn't and I walked on to the cash desk. But suddenly I thought, I've just got to have one.

Some become dominated by the thought of how much they should weigh. A lively lady of 71 talked incessantly about her love of food and concern about her weight. On occasions she gave way and ate cream and trifle and had three dry Martinis. She would still persist in constantly checking her weight. Her feelings of guilt came to the fore at every clinic check-up, which always included a weigh-in.

The interest that diabetics are encouraged to take in their bodies by checking on their weight, blood, or urine seems to contribute to an overdeveloped sense of awareness of bodily sensations (Stuart 1977).

Hypoglycaemia and hyperglycaemia

One of the major fears of insulin-dependent diabetics is of failing to achieve an appropriate blood sugar level and experiencing a 'hypo'. Hypoglycaemia is a result of having too low a level of blood glucose, too much insulin. The effects that diabetics describe when they go hypo are caused by a shortage of glucose being supplied to the brain and an increase in the body of the supply of hormones which normally produce glucose (mainly adrenalin). It has been suggested that sensations of hypos are experienced by as many as 50 per cent of insulin-dependent diabetics as frequently as once a month (Goldgewicht et al. 1983).

Many diabetics can learn to recognize the signs of an approaching hypo. Hypos develop quite quickly and are usually signalled by a tingling sensation in the lips or trembling. However, diabetics describe a range of signs. One diabetic said:

> If I'm hypo I'm very, very irritable and a very nasty person. I say things I don't mean and I rabbit on a lot, you know.

For some the initial warning of a hypo appears to vary:

> When I first had 'hypos' it was worrying as it seemed different each time. I have experienced feeling faint, dizziness and unsteadiness in walking.
>
> (*Balance* 1982: 4)

Other diabetics feel able to tell their blood sugar levels from changes in mood:

> I find if I've got a high blood sugar, I'm more quicker to anger than I am if I've got a very low blood sugar.

Hypos can occur during sleep. One mother explained the difficulty this sometimes caused her:

> My husband does shiftwork. It's not so bad of a day but of a night when I've got to go to bed on me own and I go hypo in my sleep. . . . I can't get up so if he [the baby] was choking I can't move . . .

Hypos are also associated with menstruation. A survey by Walsh (1983) reported that 30 per cent of women surveyed reported problems with their blood sugar level for as long as a week prior to their monthly period. Attacks of hyperglycaemia, too high a level of blood glucose, are experienced less frequently by diabetics. Hyperglycaemia sometimes occurs when a person is unwell, or suffers a loss of appetite and unwisely stops taking insulin. A woman who had been an insulin-dependent diabetic for thirteen years described what happened when she had a stomach upset and stopped her insulin because she was not eating:

> all through the night all I kept doing was being sick, and I was getting weaker and weaker.

It is in fact necessary for diabetics to continue with their insulin injections even though they may be suffering a loss of appetite as a result of having a cold or 'flu.

Other health problems

A less dramatic effect of the struggle to maintain a satisfactory blood sugar level is the experience of tiredness. This stems from there being insufficient insulin to assist in the process of converting glucose into energy. Tiredness is a common symptom in patients with diabetes, occurring almost twice as commonly as in non-diabetics (*Balance* 1983: 16). An insulin-dependent diabetic said:

> I find I'm terribly tired . . . you go very tired I think when you are high in sugar. . . . I often go home [from work] and sleep from four till six.

And a non-insulin-dependent woman told a similar story:

> We're always having rest . . . because sometimes, when I come in from work . . . I don't do anything, I feel so tired.

Eyesight problems resulting from retinopathy are a common complication of diabetes. Even in cases where this does not lead to blindness the resulting visual problems may be extremely handicapping. One woman who had difficulty seeing to cross roads isolated herself at home:

> As I say, my eyes are not too good. I need help everywhere so I'm better off at home.

Diabetics may also experience tingling sensations and pains in the feet, arms, and hands. These sensations may be caused either by poor circulation or by damage to the peripheral nervous system (Watkins 1984.) These may be mild symptoms:

> Of course when I get up in the morning I have all pins and needles in my hands.

Or more extreme:

> Sometimes I have a numbness here. . . . The only trouble I get is in this portion, the calf muscles. And that's bad.

Diabetes is a contributory factor in poor circulation and the direct cause of the damage to the peripheral nervous system. The numbness or loss of feeling in the feet caused by the damage to the nervous system exposes diabetics to the risk of cuts and blisters which may become infected. One woman described it as a common experience:

I get septic toes, like when I cut my toe-nails a few weeks ago,
it went all yellow colour at the corner.

A man described his injured toe more poetically:

It was, well, like seeing an oasis of blossom, like blossom on
high-speed pictures. . . . it came up all of a sudden . . . it
suddenly turned blue right down to the nail, and then it burst.

Damage to the nervous system may also cause impotence in
men. Although men are less likely to complain about it than
other effects of diabetes, a number of studies have confirmed that
impotence is commonly experienced by diabetics. Campbell and
McCulloch (1979) reported that in a sample of over 500 men aged
between 20 and 59, 35 per cent were found to have erectile
impotence. They state that: 'The usual problem is chronic impotence of gradual onset in patients who have had diabetes for some
years'.

A German study of 314 men reported that over half suffered
from sexual disturbance (Schöffling *et al.* 1963). Complex vascular
abnormalities, neuropathy, and psychological factors are involved
in the causes of impotence amongst diabetics and it has been
argued that psychological counselling is of particular importance
(Ward 1985).

The search for explanations

So far, the primary effects of the disorder have been emphasized.
But equally important are sufferers' *personal responses* to the
disorder. Many patients with diabetes or the parents of diabetics
feel the need to understand why they became diabetic. Most
search their past for an explanation. A very common source of
possible explanations is family inheritance. Others look back for
signs of greed in their eating behaviour in the past. One man said:

Well naturally it must be an excessive amount of sweetness,
sweet things that you are having. . . . I had got into the habit
of putting sugar, I like soup . . . and say I was having a bit of
vegetable soup or minestrone soup and it didn't taste quite
to my liking, I would add sugar to it you see.

A young woman remembered that at the age of 8 when she was

diagnosed she was very frightened because the sound of the word diabetes made her think she was going to die. She said she then thought it must have been punishment for being naughty and not wanting to go to school.

> I thought . . . I will go to school every day. I will behave meself from now on like. I can remember thinking it.

Many people who search their own past for an explanation of why they developed diabetes arrive at shock as being the causative factor. The shocks they describe range from being stung by an enormous bee, to being kidnapped. Diabetics, in this respect, are like many others suffering from chronic illness in both searching for an explanation and arriving at a shock as the answer. Such interpretations sharply contrast with medical opinion that, while shock may trigger the start of diabetes, it is not likely to be the underlying cause.

Some parents also blame themselves for their children's diabetes. One mother had searched for an explanation and blamed herself because she had given her 10-year-old son a good thrashing two days before he developed diabetes (Lindsay 1985.)

Fears and worries

Diabetes may be associated with various worries and concerns in relation to the present and for the long term. Concern about being overweight has already been mentioned; an insulin-dependent woman said:

> I'm putting on weight every day although I'm trying my best on the diet, I still put on weight.

For others the main worry may be loss of weight; a non-insulin-dependent woman said:

> She weigh me and she speak to me and I said to her whatever they give me to eat I don't think that can put on any weight.

A greater worry is the fear of having a hypo; many hypos occur quite unexpectedly and this results in a constant sense of uncertainty as to the timing of the next episode and how the individual will cope. One diabetic described the fear of hypos as: 'The feeling of nameless dread, the beast, is there every waking instant of my life and every night in my dreams' (McLean 1985: 116).

Another woman described how fear of having a hypo had curtailed her shopping expeditions unless she could persuade her husband to go with her:

Well it don't worry me, but it's the thought like if you go low say [in blood sugar] and you take something, for the rest of the day you feel horrible. And I just hate it happening.

Diabetics may also have worries about the future. Although some seem not to know about the risk of complications, most have some awareness that such risks exist:

If you don't look . . . take care of yourself you can possibly go blind or you can lose your legs. Some people have lost their toes. It's serious.

They may, for example, have family members who have had diabetes which resulted in complications.

Seeing other people with diabetes may alert individuals to some of the potential hazards. One diabetic woman in her 70s described how on a recent check-up visit to a hospital she had met a man she had known as fit and healthy years ago but who was now in a wheel-chair as a result of an amputation made necessary by diabetes. It had upset her for a week, she said. Another woman, an insulin-dependent diabetic, had recently spent a week in hospital, the experience of which had frightened her:

Because, as they said to me, it could be . . . you could be all right for the next ten or twenty years but it ain't now, it's when you're older – like with your legs and with your feet. I mean I was on the ward. Seeing them, legs amputated, toes amputated. It did frighten me, specially with my leg.

This fear for the future for themselves may also extend to a fear of their children developing diabetes. One woman with a 5-year-old daughter described her anxiety:

Sometimes my Mum has her [daughter] at weekends and she'll phone up and say Sue's been drinking a lot today. It's all panicky – like me and my husband get round there, do a water test [urine test]. . . . I mean you can't stop thinking of it especially when you know the signs.

Another woman described her feelings when she was told by a GP that her 18-month-old daughter was diabetic:

I came home and I said to him [husband] 'They reckon she's got diabetes'. I just couldn't look at him when I said it because I thought he's going to say to me, 'You're the one that's got it – you gave it to her', you know. And I was so scared of what he'd say.

For some young people this may be a worry even when they are at the early stages of a relationship with someone and only contemplating the responsibilities of marriage.

Case examples

Two case studies illustrate the different ways diabetes may affect people's lives.

Daisy Monk is a non-insulin-dependent diabetic who takes tablets to control her diabetes. She is aged 57 and was retired early at the age of 52 on health grounds. She had been employed as a tea-lady in a factory. At that time, and continuing to the time of interview, she had ulcers on her legs, but she had in fact been 'taken queer' at work and a blood test revealed that she was suffering from diabetes. She is overweight and has very poor eyesight. She also suffers from pins and needles in her hands. She finds the diet difficult, partly because of the expense involved in buying meat and vegetables, and partly because she says she gets contradictory advice:

they tell me not to eat potatoes and somebody else tells me to do the other thing, I mean it's one against the other, you see.

She attends a hospital out-patient clinic for check-ups and is visited once a week by a community nurse who specializes in diabetes.

Now that she is not able to work she has a very limited range of social contacts. She lives alone in a council flat which is not well-cared for. Her social contacts are the old lady next door, who insists on giving her cakes, which she says she throws away;

a woman who serves in the corner shop and who is the person she consults if she has a problem; and the nurse. She has a dog which she takes for walks round the block. Her other activities include watching the local children play, watching the television, which she cannot see very well, and listening to talking books from the library or listening to the radio. She does not go to any clubs for retired people and there is no group for diabetics in the area. She would like to go to a diabetics' group if there were one.

She regards herself as healthy and is uncomplaining about her health or the effect that having diabetes has had on her life. She is aware that diabetes can cause blindness and often makes it difficult for infections to heal. She does not spend time wondering why she got diabetes; she accepts it. Her knowledge of what causes it is confused:

Somebody said it's in your bones or something

but she also said

Well, I suppose like when you're a baby, you're fed by a bottle aren't you, and you have sugar in it, and I reckon it's probably that way, you see.

Mrs Mary Cook is an insulin-dependent diabetic aged 23. She has been diabetic for twelve years and was diagnosed after experiencing the classic symptoms of extreme thirst, vomiting, and loss of consciousness. Her GP seemed not to recognize the symptoms but when she was referred to hospital they were diagnosed immediately. No one else in her family is diabetic. For ten years she had taken her insulin injections but largely ignored any recommendations about diet:

I just ate as much as I wanted to eat

although her mother had tried to keep her to a diet. She said that she had experienced no problems with her diabetes until recently but she had, in fact, had an ulcerated leg and an infected toe which had proved difficult to heal.

At secondary school she said the teachers were over-protective and discouraged her from taking part in games. This had alerted the other children to the fact that she took injections and they began to call her a drug addict. This had upset her and she had begun truanting. When she left school she worked in a factory and that made it difficult to keep to a diet and regularly timed meals

> You've got to keep to their times; you can't keep to your times.

After working for a couple of years she got married and had a baby daughter. She and her husband worry about whether their daughter will develop diabetes. Recently she had lost another baby after a six-month pregnancy. She had then tried to start work again in a cafe but this had brought on hyperglycaemic attacks. She had spent a week in hospital and was stabilized again and now keeping carefully to the treatment regimen. She had given up her job.

She is cheerful, looking forward to having another baby, and is well supported by her husband. She has plenty of friends and sees herself as no different from them. She would not want to attend a diabetics' group if there was one nearby.

Conclusion

This chapter has described many of the wide range of symptoms that diabetics may experience. The faulty metabolism which constitutes diabetes may affect many organs and systems of the body. The diabetic may experience these effects over a long period of years, depending on how successfully and consistently a near-normal level of blood sugar is maintained. However, as salient for many sufferers are the experiential aspects of the disorder emphasized in this chapter, such as alertness to bodily symptoms, weight and diet, and concerns about the future.

Chapter three

Living with diabetic treatments

Introduction

The treatment prescribed for diabetes may be demanding and may require discipline and a willingness to make it a high priority in one's daily life. The treatment regimens, briefly described in chapter 1, are complicated schedules of controlled eating, medication in the form of insulin or tablets to stimulate the production of insulin, controlled exercise, and regular monitoring of blood glucose levels. Maintaining the correct balance of food, activity, and medication is like walking a tightrope. On one side is the danger of hypoglycaemia; on the other side hyperglycaemia. In the background is the fear of complications.

Because most aspects of daily life affect blood glucose levels, they may all have to be fitted into the treatment regimen. A regular pattern of activity with meals and snacks at planned times can be balanced by a regular amount of insulin or tablets; but unplanned activities or meals eaten later than usual require adjustments to the treatment programme. Social life is inhibited by the knowledge that taking part in unplanned activities could cause the unpleasant effects of hyperglycaemia or hypoglycaemia, and might also contribute to long-term complications. Not being able to take up social opportunities because they have not been planned for reduces spontaneity in life. Being a diabetic with a well-controlled blood sugar level means, for many people, experiencing a feeling of being controlled in another sense, that is experiencing a reduced sense of autonomy in everyday activities. There is therefore a certain irony in describing some diabetics as 'well controlled'. The diabetics' journal *Balance* often features professional sportspeople and entertainers who successfully and apparently without difficulty combine an active career with having a well-controlled blood sugar level, but for many diabetics the struggle to perform successfully their everyday roles of spouse, parent, worker, neighbour, and friend and control their blood sugar level is an enormously difficult task.

This chapter considers how the treatment regimen of diabetics intervenes in important everyday activities. It is a continual reminder to diabetics of their condition and of their difference from others. This sense of difference creates in turn a concern about being able to appear normal to others, and may involve the development of strategies to restore a sense of normality.

Insulin treatment by injections

The insulin treatment developed since Banting and Best discovered insulin in 1922 has been much improved. The insulin now used is highly purified and the means of injecting it into the body have also been improved by the development of disposable syringes and needles, injector guns, and more recently an infusion pump which eliminates the need for injections. Different types of insulin have been developed which remain active for varying lengths of time after being injected. These are all improvements in terms of regulating the level of blood sugar, but they also require the diabetic to possess a greater knowledge of how injected insulin works.

Injected insulin is used in the body differently from the way naturally produced insulin is used. Naturally occurring insulin is not produced in sudden large amounts. It is supplied on demand to maintain a more or less constant level of glucose in the blood. When an amount of insulin is injected it quickly becomes active in the bloodstream and starts to lower the level of blood sugar; it goes on reducing the level until it has been used up and it may drastically reduce the level of glucose until a hypo is experienced. For this reason the amount of insulin injected has to be carefully calculated and measured. In order to reduce the problem of suddenly increasing the level of insulin in the blood from an injection, several different types of insulin have been developed, varying in terms of the speed with which they act. Normal soluble insulin acts rapidly, but its action can be slowed to varying degrees. Insulin-dependent diabetics therefore need to know which types of insulin they are using. The complexity of insulin regime faced by some diabetics is illustrated by one sufferer:

> I've got an ultra-tard which lasts for about thirty-six hours [very slow acting] and makes a background, and then I have insula-tard in the morning which lasts about twelve hours [slow acting], I think, a bit less than that. And I have act-rapid in the evening.

Without this kind of knowledge they cannot accommodate changes in the pattern of their activities. If a diabetic is going to engage in strenuous physical activity such as playing football or tennis, for example, it might be necessary to reduce the amount of quick-acting insulin injected before playing. Insulin-dependent diabetics on shiftwork also have to make adjustments to their treatment regimen as their pattern of meals and physical activity change.

The timing of injections also requires careful attention. Normally an injection is given just before a meal so that the insulin is available in the bloodstream when required for the metabolic processes which make use of food as glucose. If a meal is delayed, however, the insulin will start acting and reduce the blood sugar level before more glucose becomes available. The unpleasant feelings of a 'hypo' will then start to develop. Having to time injections in relation to eating is one of the worries that diabetics have in relation to eating out, or being in social situations where it is difficult to insist that meals arrive at the right time. One diabetic described her situation at a dinner party at which the hostess, for a long while, provided only nibbles of toast and fish instead of the substantial meal that she had planned for and injected for (McLean 1985). When the main courses finally arrived she wolfed hers down and was embarrassed to see the disapproving glances of other guests.

The need for insulin is reduced during sleep as the body is inactive and no food is taken in. The evening injection of insulin has to be carefully calculated to be sufficient to metabolize the evening meal and to prevent hyperglycaemia developing, but not enough to cause a night-time hypo. Nocturnal hypos are not uncommon and although some people sleep through them, other diabetics have experienced nightmares; others wake early with the unpleasant feeling still with them.

Managing to achieve a comfortable blood sugar level throughout the day and night requires insulin-dependent diabetics to have knowledge of how insulin works, a willingness to monitor blood sugar levels, and the determination to check other factors in the equation that may achieve balance, food, and activity. Those who do achieve a satisfactory balance often acknowledge the support of a husband or wife. Fletcher (1982: 79) attributes his successful management of forty years of diabetes to the help he has received from his wife and her ability to recognize the signs of a hypo.

> Once I clutched my wife saying, 'The world is coming to an end, and I want to hold on to you'. 'All right,' she said, 'but drink some Lucozade first', and the world was saved.

Teenage diabetics find the discipline and responsibility of balancing insulin injections, eating, and exercise particularly difficult to manage. At this stage in their lives they are very involved with peer-group activities and they are making new relationships which may seem more important than anything else. Eating meals at regular times and timing injections seem a hindrance to social life. A teenage girl attending a further education college explained her problem:

> I couldn't stay at college and go straight to netball. I had to rush home first and then rush back. They did suggest taking it [insulin] to college with me but I felt a bit of an idiot.

Joining in activities and living in a carefree way is an important part of being like other teenagers. The attraction of joining in peer-group activities spontaneously not only makes it difficult to eat regularly and relate eating to injections and activity but also creates conflicts with caring parents.

> My dad has a go at me. 'Are you eating the right food?' But I just don't take no notice of him.

The parents of teenage diabetics have not only the usual problems associated with allowing their children a growing amount of independence, but also the added problems of trying to prevent them from harming themselves by neglecting their diabetes (Lindsay

1985). Teenagers may come to feel that having diabetes places too much responsibility on them at an early age (Sullivan 1979) and may develop a sense of resentment because of their parents' reluctantance to allow them independence from the family.

The act of having to inject oneself initially scares many diabetics and some are also worried about their ability to measure and inject the correct amount. A few diabetics never lose this fear of injecting. Those who become diabetic in middle age and who do not respond to treatment by tablets often find injecting distressing. One diabetic woman who had been on tablets but was now on insulin said:

> I manage to do it now, but I don't feel all right with it. But I still manage to do it, and worst of all two times a day, which is so difficult.

Others dislike it but adopt a more stoic approach.

> Sometimes I sort of grind me teeth, you know, but it's got to be done.

Others clearly do get used to the experience. They describe it as a daily routine as familiar as cleaning their teeth.

> Some mornings I've done it and I can't remember doing it. . . . I've had to feel me arm to feel the insulin, you know, in case I forgot.

Another problem associated with injections is finding suitable sites on the body. Just how commonly experienced a problem it is is shown by the frequent references to it in the correspondence columns of *Balance* (the British Diabetics Association journal). Many people inject into their thighs, but some use their arms, or stomach, and some use their calf if it is easier during the day (Fletcher 1982). Doctors advise diabetics to vary the site they use both to avoid the appearance of lumps in the flesh and because when lumps appear the insulin is then likely to be absorbed more slowly and unpredictably. Even diabetics who have grown used to injecting find that there are some places in their body into which they cannot bring themselves to inject.

> It don't bother me doing it but it would be nice . . . like to give me arms a rest. I can't do it in me thighs, I dunno why, I just can't. I can't do it in me stomach, so it's just me arms.

Because diabetes often requires frequent injections in the course of the day, there will often be occasions when finding a suitable social location in which to inject may present a problem. Diabetics often avoid injecting themselves in public for fear of embarrassment to themselves or others. Indeed some diabetics fear being mistaken for drug addicts (Hopper 1981). One obvious place to use is a public lavatory, but these may be full or filthy. The choice then facing the diabetic is either to inject furtively or to resort to injecting in front of embarrassed strangers (McLean 1985). This makes diabetes a more public affair than many diabetics may wish.

Taking tablets

Nearly half of non-insulin-dependent diabetics take tablets to help control their diabetes. The tablets are prescribed in conjunction with a diet and are taken just before meals. It is not important for non-insulin-dependent diabetics to take their meals and tablets at the same time each day, and their treatment routine is therefore more flexible than that of insulin-dependent diabetics but even with this flexibility, the taking of tablets still presents problems for some. One man who rose very early in the morning in order to work in a vegetable market did not have time for breakfast and so missed his morning tablet altogether.

> I found I didn't want to take it of a morning because I didn't have a very full meal and tend to sort of . . . I don't eat properly during the day really . . . I thought to myself, I won't take it in the mornings, I'll only take it in the evenings.

Taking tablets in the morning would have meant having breakfast, and that would have interfered with his work routine; for him work was more important than his diabetes.

The use of tablets which stimulate the production of natural insulin and are long acting create their own difficulties. If, having taken a tablet, one forgets to eat or does not feel like eating for a day or so, there is the danger of an oversupply of insulin and the possibility of a hypo (Lebovitz 1985).

Monitoring blood glucose levels

Measuring the amount of glucose in the urine or blood is an important part of the process of achieving a balance between food eaten, activity engaged in, and the need for insulin. Monitoring the level of glucose in the blood needs to be done two or three times a day to provide necessary feedback information to the diabetic and is especially important for those attempting to achieve normoglycaemia. This information can be used to make appropriate adjustments to the insulin dosage, the food intake, or the amount of physical activity engaged in. The blood test is the more direct and accurate measure as the level at which glucose appears in the urine varies from individual to individual. At the moment in Britain diabetics are not supplied with a meter for blood tests through the NHS so many continue with urine tests.

Diabetics sometimes maintain that they can tell from how they feel whether their blood sugar level is high or low.

> How I feel inside, how I feel when I move, when I walk. If I've got a high blood sugar I get to the top of the turning and I've got pains in me legs.

Most doctors are sceptical about the ability of diabetics to know sufficiently accurately whether their blood sugar level is high or low, but there is evidence that, with training, diabetics might be able to estimate their own blood sugar levels by attending to cues from physical symptoms or mood states (Bradley 1985).

Some diabetics assume that as long as they feel well their blood sugar level must be within reasonable limits. They test only when they feel unwell:

> I do it now and again, when I feel I'm a bit ill.

or

> If I feel lousy, you know, I think I've got a bad migraine coming on, straight away I test the blood sugar.

Monitoring blood sugar levels is a part of the treatment routine which is confusing to some diabetics and disliked by many. As many as 25 per cent of diabetics may be unsure of what to do with test results (Mason 1985). Some do not test their blood sugar levels because they do not know how to use the information.

Well if it's high, I don't know what to do, honestly, I just don't know what to do.

It may simply become painful to keep pricking a finger for a blood sample:

I mean for four years I've been doing them. My fingers and toes are so sore. They told me not to use my toes, you know, but I ran out of fingers, I had to use my toes.

Other people just forget to monitor regularly:

I only do it sometimes, when I remember.

The intrusive nature of some recommendations is evidenced by one diabetic who said she tried to follow the treatment regimen but drew the line when it was suggested to her that she should check her blood sugar level before engaging in 'extra-curricular activity' after bedtime (*Balance*, 1985).

Having to monitor blood sugar levels may also be disliked by many diabetics because it may provide frustrating evidence of their failure to control their illness in spite of attempts to follow the treatment regimen. It may also provide an unpleasant reminder of the potential long-term consequences of the illness (Hauser and Polletts 1979; Tattersall and Jackson 1982).

For a minority of diabetics monitoring provides information which allows them to achieve a sense of control over their illness. Some keep detailed charts of the results of their testing to show to the doctor at their next clinic appointment. This sense of control leads them to a more general confidence that they can act independently of health professionals:

I'm decreasing and increasing it [insulin] how I feel I should and that's what they want you to do. And I'd rather leave it to me than keep getting on the phone all the time saying, 'What do I do?'

Although monitoring does give diabetics feedback on how they are managing their diabetes, it is useful only if they do it sufficiently often and take appropriate action either on their own understanding or after consulting with the nurse or doctor (Tattersall 1985).

Some diabetics who fail to do regular monitoring of their blood sugar level feel guilty about it. Rather than admit their failure to the doctor they resort to producing faked records of tests. Until recently doctors were unable to challenge diabetics' claims that their blood sugar level had been well controlled. Recently, however, a new test of blood sugar level has been developed. The glycosylated haemoglobin or HbA1 measure will show the average level of blood glucose over the previous two or three months. Although some diabetics may see the use of this test as 'policing' it provides doctors with valuable and reliable information.

Dietary control

Diet is an important consideration for all diabetics. On the one hand the timing of food is important in order to maintain a balanced blood sugar level. On the other hand, weight control is important because of the risks associated with obesity, and this requires careful attention to both the amount and types of food eaten. For insulin-dependent diabetics the timing of meals (and injections) is an additional and critical concern.

Until 1983 (British Diabetic Association 1983) the kind of diet recommended for diabetics was a low carbohydrate one with foods like bread, potatoes, cereals, and sugar being strictly limited. Diabetics were provided with a list of foods they could eat. The list also told them some of the exchanges they could make in their diet, for example one portion of potato could be exchanged or replaced in a meal by, say, one slice of bread or two tablespoons of yams, or an ice-cream could be exchanged for fifteen strawberries. The exchange list gave diabetics the freedom to vary their diet provided they were able and willing to study their food intake in this way. It also enabled them to work out a number of standard meals which they could eat without thinking too much about their diet.

The dietary recommendations of the BDA were changed in Britain in 1983 as epidemiological evidence had suggested that control of the energy value of diet was perhaps more appropriate than the control of carbohydrate intake. The changed aim of dietary control also made it possible for diabetics to be advised to eat the same type of low fat, high fibre diet currently thought of as a healthy diet for the general population. Diabetics do however have to know the energy value of the foods they eat and ration themselves according to their diet sheets. Foods can still be exchanged for other foods of the same energy value, but calculating the exchanges remains a problem for many diabetics.

Some attempt to avoid the calculations by restricting themselves to a very limited range of foods, which makes for a monotonous diet. The diet is more difficult for diabetics controlled by tablets and diet than it is for those using insulin. Those on insulin have another factor in the equation which they can manipulate. If they eat too much they can adjust their insulin.

> If you are going out to eat and drink . . . I put my insulin up and I don't eat my evening meal [at home].

Those whose diabetes is controlled by diet and tablets have no such way out. An elderly woman said she had kept to the same diet for the last twenty-four years.

> I don't buy anything I mustn't have.

She did not go out to eat because

> I mean, if you go anywhere, sticking to a diet is hard outside; indoors I know just where I am.

Many diabetics come to rely on a narrow range of foods that they feel sure of rather than rely on the more varied but also more complex dietary regimen encouraged by dieticians. Another elderly woman was restricted in another way. She did go out but kept to a restricted range of foods:

> Well, if I go out I'll only have a salad. I wouldn't, I don't have anything else. I have a salad or steamed fish but I won't have anything else.

Some diabetics develop their own criteria of 'acceptable' and 'unacceptable' food, which may often be excessively restrictive. One diabetic ate just cabbage, carrots, lettuce, and tomatoes at home and took his own home-made sandwiches to work. His interpretation of the dietary recommendations had led him to a restricted range of foods, mainly vegetables.

Others keep strictly to recommended diets and manage to eat more interestingly. A 76-year-old retired man took great care over what he ate. He had studied his diet sheet carefully:

> Yes so I myself, I watch me food. Mind you I eat well. Oh, I

have a lovely dinner. But I've read this [diet sheet] a
thousand times to see if I'm going over the amounts.

In a few cases, the calculations involved in controlling diet become
a time-consuming activity, indeed a preoccupation. A young
woman who was insulin-dependent meticulously observed her
diet:

Like two scoops of potatoes, 20 grammes and all that, you
know. A slice of bread 10 grammes. . . . You literally eat
the same as them [the rest of the family] but it's less
amounts. . . . I can only have two tablespoons of peas.

There are two ways in which dietary control may break down.
For some the temptations of proscribed foods are too great. Those
living on low wages or social security have a very different
problem; the expense involved in eating special food, different
from the rest of the family, places too great a strain on the meagre
budget. As one diabetic succinctly described the problem:

They [Social Security] only allow me 50p a week for the diet,
you know.

Concern about weight and eating correctly is a central part of the
experience of being diabetic for non-insulin-dependent diabetics.
It is a concern which clouds their enjoyment of food, one of the
pleasures of life, and also inhibits social life. Insulin-dependent
diabetics are also concerned with not exceeding the prescribed
amount of food but if they are going to over-eat many of them
simply adjust the amount of insulin to cope with the increased
need they anticipate.

Treatment involves adjustments to meals, injections, tablet-
taking, and testing blood sugar levels; such requirements are
demanding and invasive so that other considerations have to be
fitted around them. This reduced flexibility in social arrangements
leads to diabetics not being able to respond to unexpected invi-
tations. Apparently simple decisions such as to go for a drink with
friends or to go further afield than planned for on a shopping trip
become matters to be considered rather than acted on spontaneously. To some such restrictions create a feeling of being
completely dominated by their diabetes:

> I think it [diabetes] rules your life. Other people say they don't think it does, they are able to forget about it, but I can't.

Coping with diabetes

Coping is a term widely used in the literature of chronic illness and disability. Although it has been used differently by different authors, one common theme is that chronic illnesses involve both emotional and practical problems which have to be dealt with. How people cope may be influenced by their social environment, by their personal characteristics, and most importantly by the particular ways in which they perceive and evaluate problems. The concept of appraisal (Folkman and Lazarus 1980) is important in that it draws attention to such perceptions and evaluations.

People perceive and evaluate the demands of diabetic treatment very differently. Some see the demands of the regimen in practical terms. The problems, to them, are those of achieving a satisfactory level of blood sugar, not going hypo, and accommodating the treatment regimen to other important aspects of living, such as work, social life, or shopping and looking after a family. Thus the demands of the treatment regimen are perceived as practical problems requiring practical solutions. When the problem is seen as one of timing injections so that other activities can be continued, then practical arrangements can be made to have meals and injections at conveniently altered times and the dosage of insulin can be altered if necessary. As one diabetic explained.

> I can live the life I want to live more or less. If I'm going out for a booze, or if I'm going out to a dinner and dance, I make it [the amount of insulin injected] according to what I am eating and drinking.

When things go wrong, they may be seen as the result of practical problems which could be put right by making practical adjustments. A young woman with two young children to look after said the problems she experienced were caused by her inability to fit in snacks between meals.

> Lack of food, definitely. I don't eat enough. It's only because I say I haven't got time, which is true, I haven't. I just haven't got the time to keep sitting down eating.

Another respondent, who at the age of 76 still led a physically very active life, described his way of coping in very practical terms.

> I haven't took a test this morning but if I take the test now see, I find that it's negative. I have me dinner and after midday, say in the evening, I take another test. . . . I'd always find that it would go up after I'd been eating see . . . so it proves that dieting is the right thing.

Problems are defined and responses directed to a practical solution. This practical approach may also give the individual a sense of autonomy, a feeling of being in control rather than controlled by diabetes and by the demands of the treatment regimen. Furthermore, viewing diabetes in this way may also help to avoid the feelings of being different that are behind some sufferers' sense of stigma. One diabetic expressed her feelings as

> I'm the same as the next. You know what I mean? I class myself the same as everyone else, even though I take injections.

Others, however, view their treatment as creating wider problems. They may feel that their everyday life is so transformed as a result of their treatment regimen that they feel cursed with a serious illness which marks them out as different from others as well as from their former selves. Although diabetes is a disease which is not directly visible to others, there are various ways in which it may become public. The problems of injecting in public have already been mentioned. Sufferers may have to restrict their food when eating socially. Another important part of the treatment regimen may be a weight-reducing diet. However, this treatment also alters their appearance. This public aspect of the disease makes it difficult for some to treat it as a practical problem.

> You see when people go on that strict diet it makes you look like, terrible. People say, 'Oh, what's wrong with you? . . . Is it you?'

The overall effect of losing weight may please the doctor but present the diabetic with fresh problems with regard to appearance and self-image. Diabetes is something many sufferers want to conceal:

> I don't want anybody to know. I don't want anybody to know I'm diabetic and all that. I feel embarrassed.

However, the personal sense of being different may become a pervasive and distressing dimension of the illness. For some, the very idea of having an illness, such as diabetes, leads them to hold a diminished view of themselves. One diabetic who previously had prided himself on his fitness and his capacity to go on long-distance road walks, admitted that he was under pressure to change his view of himself. His mother was insisting that he should take things more easily because of his health:

> She's trying to get it instilled into me that I can't do what I could do, and I have to slow down. Which I feel I do agree with in one way.

His reservations arose from difficulties in accepting a view of himself as 'weak'.

Such threats to individuals' sense of self are distressing and may give rise to 'coping strategies' rather than the practical problem-solving approach. One such coping strategy can be described as avoidance, when diabetics attempt to minimize the emotional threat and uncertainties about their identity by avoiding social situations which present them with difficulties. Not eating out, not eating at other people's homes, reducing social activities generally, become not so much ways of keeping to the treatment regimen by avoiding temptation, but rather part of a strategy to keep diabetes invisible to others.

Another strategy is to reduce the importance attached to any symptoms of diabetes, that is a 'minimizing' strategy, where symptoms come to be seen not as a threat but as a normal part of having diabetes. A diabetic who adopted this strategy explained that during the daytime when he was working he restricted his drinking to one bottle of water that he took with him, but at home in the evening he drank a great deal, with the result that he had to go to the lavatory several times each night. He accepted this: as he saw things, it was a normal part of having diabetes.

> You can't have the 'flu without sneezing.

The concept of normalization has been used by a number of social scientists to refer to ways by which disabled people structure situations to make their disability less obvious to others (Davis 1961; 1963; Haber and Smith 1971; Strauss and Glaser 1975; Weiner 1975). The strategies of social avoidance and of mini-mizing are particular ways in which some diabetics normalize otherwise distressing aspects of life created by their treatment regimen. Normalization may reduce the emotional stress when the demands of the diabetic treatment regimen are experienced as a threat to identity, and may promote a more general sense of well-being as it allows feelings of being different from others to be pushed backstage (Kelleher forthcoming).

Another response to treatment is one of worry, anxiety, and depression in relation to the disorder (Treuting 1961; Murawski *et al*. 1970). A diabetic woman who also had arthritis described her distressing feelings:

> I take tablets for the arthritis but it doesn't get rid of the pain . . . but I still think the diabetes is worse. . . . Because it could cause complications, couldn't it.

Another woman complained of always feeling tired and of numerous aches and pains that she attributed to her diabetes and this made her depressed:

> Sometimes I'm sitting here and I'm depressed, but it's not because I'm depressed, it's knowing that I have it [diabetes].

For others the depression is more extreme:

> I can sit here now with the family and not say one word some days, just sit there with the hump for no reason at all.

For some patients their depressed mood is clearly a direct response to the diabetes. For others, however, this response may be to the indirect social consequences of diabetes, such as unemployment (Fris and Nanjundappa (1986)).

Personality and response to treatment

The early observations of Willis in 1697 and Maudsley in 1899 noted the frequent presence of 'prolonged sorrow' in the life histories of people who became diabetic. It certainly seems likely that different personalities will respond differently to having diabetes and to the treatment regimens or what has been called 'the tyranny of metabolic manipulation' (Dunn and Turtle 1981: 644). The difficulty is in choosing an appropriate typology of personalities.

One useful method uses the locus of control concept (Rotter 1966), which suggests that while some people see the things that happen to them as being the result of their own skill and effort (internal locus of control), others are more likely to regard events as the result of forces independent of their control (external locus of control). One study of insulin-dependent diabetics showed that those who preferred to have an insulin pump rather than injections tended to have an external locus of control (Bradley *et al.* 1984). This suggests that diabetic people with an external locus of control may be unsuitable patients to be fitted with a subcutaneous pump. A diabetic fitted with a pump has to be more than usually careful in regularly monitoring his blood sugar level, so that more responsibility is placed on the patient, not less. However there is no conclusive evidence that people with an internal locus of control do manage to control their blood sugar levels more effectively (Bradley 1985).

From time to time it has been hypothesized that having diabetes affects personality in a general way and leads to the development of a 'diabetic personality' (Benedek 1948). The evidence to support this hypothesis has not been forthcoming (Hauser and Polletts 1979; Dunn and Turtle 1981).

Conclusion

It has been suggested in a medical textbook that the aim of treatment for diabetics

> is to achieve for the patient, as far as possible a state of health which is taken for granted and seldom intrudes into consciousness. Obviously this is not too difficult when a restricted diet is all that is needed.
>
> (Malins 1968: 448)

This chapter has suggested that achieving a 'state of health which is taken for granted' is not something which is easily accomplished, even when the treatment regimen is a restricted diet alone. The social-psychological problems created by diabetic treatments should be recognized by health professionals, because keeping to such demanding treatment requirements frequently proves too difficult for many patients.

Chapter four

Compliance and non-compliance

Introduction

This chapter looks at the extent to which patients follow the therapeutic advice they are given and explores the explanations for non-compliance. Several studies have shown that non-compliance is common amongst people suffering from chronic illness (Sackett and Haynes 1976; Cerkoney and Hart 1980; Hopper 1981; Ley 1982). Becker and Maiman (1980: 113) describe the general situation:

> Depending upon the characteristics of the condition, the treatment, the patient and the setting, estimates of non-compliance rates typically range from thirty per cent to sixty per cent, and the situation worsens markedly where the patients are symptom free.

Some authorities regard non-compliance as the most serious problem facing medical practice today (Becker and Maiman 1980) and diabetics appear to be at least as non-compliant as other people with chronic illness. Diabetic patients are expected to comply with instructions about diet, medication, and monitoring.

Some prefer to talk of adhering to the treatment regimen, rather than compliance, because adherence seems to convey better the self-regulatory requirements of the diabetic regimen (Brownlee-Duffeck et al. 1987: 139). Others refer to patients and doctors collaborating in the therapeutic alliance, which underlines the potential value of equal partnership between doctor and patient in resolving health problems. However it is expressed, the concern is that the patients should follow the instructions they are given in order that the condition being treated is improved. Most doctors treating diabetic patients would agree that:

the success of long-term maintenance therapy for diabetes . . .
depends largely on the extent to which the patient's
behaviour coincides with clinical prescriptions.

(Cerkoney and Hart 1980: 594)

Compliance for diabetics does not simply mean attending regularly at clinics and taking the prescribed tablets or insulin. Non-insulin-dependent diabetics are usually on a weight-reducing diet and are required to monitor their blood sugar level by regularly testing their blood or urine; many will be taking tablets. Insulin-dependent diabetics have to balance their food intake with their level of physical activity and amount of insulin injected, and their injections have to be carefully timed to precede meals; they also have to monitor their blood sugar levels.

Being compliant therefore means that diabetics have to make changes in their life-style. The difficulties in complying stem only partly from the problems of administering insulin or remembering to take tablets; compliance also requires interference in what are often long-established social customs of eating and drinking. The disruption and control of these activities, which are important social rituals in which relationships are developed and identities sustained, cause difficulties for many diabetics. Another aspect of the treatment regimen which is disliked by many diabetics, and is therefore subject to non-compliance, is the monitoring of blood sugar levels. Testing one's urine is unpleasant and pricking a finger for a blood test can be a nuisance. Monitoring and recording test results also remind people that they are diabetic and the results of tests may present them with problems they do not want to confront. Given the wide range of responsibilities expected of diabetics, it is not surprising that patients selectively comply with some aspects of the treatment regimen but not with others (Schafer *et al.* 1983.)

The assessment of compliance

All studies of compliance have their limitations. Self-reports by patients are likely to overestimate compliance and patients under observation may behave differently from when they are not being observed. Outcome measures, such as changes in weight or HbA1 tests of blood sugar level, may not be accurate measures of compliance either, as physiological factors may affect blood sugar level independently of behaviour. But all studies of non-compliance amongst diabetics confirm the small percentage who comply totally (Surwit, Scovern, and Feinglos 1982). A sample of thirty diabetics of whom twenty-one were treated with insulin revealed that 7 per cent were completely compliant (Cerkoney and Hart 1980).

In general compliance rates are highest in relation to the administration of insulin. Failure to take insulin would, for insulin-dependent diabetics, soon produce the severe and serious symptoms of hyperglycaemia, of course. Insulin-dependent diabetics, though, may not follow medical advice about how much insulin to inject and when to inject. They may be casual in measuring and administering insulin or they may not time injections properly. A woman who had been an insulin-dependent diabetic for sixteen years still hated the thought of being ruled by diabetes:

> I don't eat straight after my insulin, which you should do. I
> really do think diabetics should eat after their insulin for
> their own sake. But I can't, I can't bring myself to eat then
> because I feel that I'm trapped.

One reason for not complying is therefore a desire to avoid the sense of being controlled by the disorder. Another reason for non-compliance may be a more relaxed strategy about following medical instructions. A man who had been diabetic for eighteen years also made sure that he took his insulin but admitted to guessing how much he needed.

> If I am going out for a dinner and dance I make it according
> to what I'm eating and drinking. . . . I know roughly what
> I'm going to eat, what I'm going to drink, and roughly how
> much insulin I need to counteract that.

This respondent illustrates another way in which patients' decisions may diverge from their medical advice. Patients may come to exercise considerable independent judgement about their treatment regimes. What appears to the doctor as non-compliance is in fact a different agenda that the patient brings to treatment. The above patient said that he had once found that the kind of insulin he had been given did not suit him, so he reverted to a previous type:

I didn't tell them [doctors]. I got me old insulin out, I go back to that.

Another major reason for non-adherence across the range of requirements for diabetics is that patients may not fully understand or master the tasks that are expected. Watkin *et al.* (1967) found that out of a sample of sixty diabetics 80 per cent did not administer their insulin correctly. Another study (Hulka *et al.* 1976) showed that patients' errors in administering their insulin was a frequent cause of non-compliance.

The monitoring of blood sugar levels indicates whether any changes need to be made to the insulin dosage, but is a part of the treatment regimen which is often not done regularly. In the study by Watkin and colleagues (1967) it was reported that 45 per cent of the sample did not monitor their blood sugar level adequately, and other studies have produced similar evidence of non-compliance in respect of monitoring (Gabriele and Marble 1949). Bodansky (1986) argues that a discussion of a patient's record of monitoring of blood sugar level is an integral part of a consultation in a diabetic clinic, but when he asked one hundred diabetics to produce their records fifty-nine of them were unable to do so.

The part of the treatment regimen where there is least compliance is the diet. Early studies by Watkin *et al.* (1967) and Tunbridge and Weatherill (1970) recorded a high proportion of non-compliance with diet. The latter study was an observation-based study and it was noted that only sixteen out of a sample of ninety-four kept closely to their diet. Hopper (1981) reported from a study of low-income diabetics that fewer than one in ten patients were compliant and that 'the major issue of conflict was related to obesity and the failure to follow the diabetic diet'. West (1973), using weight change as an outcome measure of compliance with diet, reported that in a large sample of non-insulin-dependent diabetics their mean weight had increased rather than decreased after four and a half years of diet. Since one of the aims of the diet for these patients had been to reduce weight, their increase in weight was taken as an indication of their non-compliance.

Many diabetics admit to 'cheating' a little with their diet. As one 17-year-old said:

> Well, when I'm passing cake shops. . . . Sometimes I have a quick look . . . I have the odd little thing, cheat sometimes.

Others adopt a freer approach; an insulin-dependent diabetic said:

> I went to see the dietitian once and they said to me, how many grammes are you on a day? I went well, none, you know. Because as I say, I used to eat what I wanted.

A young diabetic man who lived a free-and-easy bachelor life said:

> I'll have steak, egg, and chips here at say six o'clock, I'll go out and have a few beers – that makes me hungry so I'll go to the Chinese and get spare ribs, Special Chow Mein, a piece of roast duck, come back here and me and the dog will eat it between us.

Explanations of non-compliance

Non-compliance does not necessarily mean that patients are wilful or lacking in self-control; sometimes treatment conflicts with working routines which make it difficult to have meals and injections at the same time each day. A teacher described how she found the irregular hours of work in a college of further education disrupted any efforts at regularizing her treatment and monitoring:

> I found when I was in further education that it was impossible. I was working sometimes from nine am until nine at night. And I'd have another afternoon where I'd not have to go in. I found that impossible and, in fact, I left further education for that reason.

The diabetic wife of a shiftworker explained how her husband's changing hours of work and her own need for meals at regular times created problems:

> Sunday is a very awkward day, because, as I said, my husband being a nightworker, if he's working say Saturday night and he doesn't get to bed till Sunday morning, I leave my injection a bit later to what I normally have it during the week. So it

means I have to have my meals later through the day . . . I have to jiggle it about.

Others explain that the diet or its effects conflict with their long-held, culturally based views about food. Patients may have different beliefs from their doctor about their ideal body weight and the need to diet:

Sometimes I feel I do need a little bit of sweet, of energy, things to give me energy sometimes.

Some regard food as a necessary fuel that contributes to health and to feelings of well-being. Others do not like to lose too much weight: perhaps their husbands like them to be 'well-covered', not thin:

He said to me I'm getting skinny . . . and I don't like him telling me that.

The non-compliance of these people in respect of their diet is not simply a failure to resist temptation but is more the result of feeling cross-pressured. The doctor and dietitian tell them to control their eating to lose weight, but social and cultural factors encourage them to eat more generously.

The Health Belief Model (Becker 1974) attempts formally to bring together a variety of different perceptions and beliefs about health and illness which may explain important behaviours such as compliance. The model predicts that compliance is likely to be dependent on four factors: (1) patients' level of interest in health matters in general, (2) views of how vulnerable they are to the relevant disease and its complications, (3) perceptions of the seriousness of the disease they have, and (4) their evaluations of the costs and benefits of adhering to treatment regimens. A number of studies applying this model to diabetes have shown that the belief which correlates most highly with people being compliant tends to be the belief that their diabetes is a serious illness (Cerkoney and Hart 1980; Alogna 1980). In the Alogna study it was reported that those who were rated as compliant believed that their diabetes was serious even though they had no more evidence of complications than those in the non-compliance group. A later study (Brownlee-Duffeck *et al.* 1987) suggested that compliance might be related to different beliefs according to age. For compliant older patients the most important health belief was that treatment was beneficial; younger patients were more likely to be compliant if they perceived the condition as serious and saw themselves as susceptible.

If this finding has general applicability, to what extent should health professionals present diabetes as a serious disease in order to achieve compliance? If diabetes is described as 'mild' and the risk of complications are not emphasized, patients may well not bother very much about compliance with the treatment regimen. They may feel like one woman who, although she had poor eyesight, had failed to comply with the treatment regimen and had done little to reduce her weight of 15½ stones. She said:

> I don't regard it as an illness. I don't think it's an illness, I don't know. It's not like cancer or that kind of illness.

If the seriousness of the illness is emphasized, by reference for example to the possibility of amputation of a limb, blindness, kidney failure, or heart disease, patients may well react by becoming dispirited. One woman whose condition had worsened even though she had tried hard to comply with the treatment regimen found it difficult to talk about her diabetes without getting upset. There was no doubt in her mind about how serious it was:

> It is worse than TB, it is incurable unless God helps the doctors to find out more about it. . . . I pray one day that will happen.

Although differences between patients' beliefs about their condition do not explain everything about non-compliance, the Health Belief Model does suggest that non-compliance may be intentional in the sense that patients weigh up the costs and benefits of complying with treatment by reference not only to their individual beliefs about health but also to other valued aspects of their life-style. Their ideas of 'normal' eating and drinking will be shaped by the patterns of social interaction important in their lives.

Controlling diet and the consumption of alcohol for health reasons often fit more easily into a middle-class life-style than a working-class one (Drummond 1985). In particular the demands of working-class jobs may necessitate more compromises with treatment regimens. A lorry driver's mate described how much he had to adjust his diet to the demands of his work:

Sometimes I've had an injection at six in the morning and I haven't had me breakfast until quarter to twelve. Mind you I ate a Mars bar or shifted a cake like. I've said to the lorry driver, pull over there, I'm starving and I'll get a doughnut.

Domestic responsibilities may also interfere with compliance:

I'll get up in the morning and the first thing I do is put my kettle on, have my insulin, and make a cup of tea . . . then feed the baby, then after that it's a rush to get her [other child] to the nursery.

The concept of brittle diabetes has been used to describe those diabetics whose blood sugar level oscillates between being very high and very low; this may arise as a special case of intentional non-compliance. A study by Gill *et al.* (1985) describes thirty-three case of brittle diabetes. While some were caused by hormonal changes or recurrent infections, in others the brittleness was engineered by the patient. The authors suggest that many of their patients had a 'Micawber-like' serenity about their diabetes and also seemed to create periods of being out of control, in terms of blood sugar levels, in order to gain admittance to hospital and so escape from an intolerable home situation for a while.

Complying with a diabetic treatment regimen and matching food intake and physical activity with insulin medication is a finely judged balance and it is of course easy to make genuine mistakes; however diabetics may deliberately get it wrong in order to produce symptoms and obtain help and sympathy. The sick-role is always available as a retreat, and the pathway to it can be by non-compliance (Tattersall and Walford 1985).

The intentional non-compliance of brittle diabetics is, however, only a small part of non-compliance, and it is the larger group of non-compliants that most need to be understood. Other concepts need to be developed for this purpose, for example 'role'. Individuals have numerous responsibilities and expectations placed upon them as spouses, parents, workers, and friends; chronically ill people also have further responsibilities which may be seen as an additional role. People have to attach priorities to these various roles and expectations, and non-compliance may be considered the rational outcome of evaluating such personal priorities. What remains unclear at present and warrants further research is whether certain roles are more associated with non-compliance.

This way of looking at non-compliance needs to be linked to the earlier discussion of coping strategies used by diabetics. Many diabetics manage their diabetes by normalizing, restricting their social activities to situations in which their diabetes is not apparent to others, and by keeping to their diet only so long as it does not interfere with valued activities such as work. Any symptoms which re-occur as result of non-compliance are tolerated as being part of the cost of retaining a 'normal' identity. For some diabetics, therefore, a higher priority may be attached to normalization than to adherence to treatment regimens.

Considered in this way non-compliance may be the result of a rational process of weighing up the costs and benefits of medical advice, which suggests that in the medical consultation many diabetics carefully evaluate whether advice is valuable or whether treatment proves effective. A young woman explained her priorities.

> I mean, I know that when I get to 70 or 60, or even 50, I'll go blind. I know I will. Or my leg will play up, you know. Because I abuse my diabetes. But as I said, at least them fifty or seventy years I'm going to live happy. I'm not going to sort of say, oh I can't go shopping now because I've got to have [something to eat]. I just couldn't cope with it.

She did not disbelieve medical advice and she was not unaware of some of the likely consequences of her partial compliance, but she chose to manage her diabetes according to her own priorities at that time. Chronically ill people such as diabetics may see their illness quite differently from their doctors.

The locus of control construct, discussed on p. 42, may have specific value in predicting compliance. Wierenga (1980) reported a positive link between compliance and an internal locus of control. There are clearly problems however with the construct (Nagy and Wolfe 1984); it is unclear whether individuals with internal or external locus of control are more likely to comply with medical advice. While an individual with internal locus of control may be self-motivated, those with an external locus of control may religiously follow the doctor's advice. Both approaches might be considered to produce high levels of adherence to long-term treatment regimens, and so we should distinguish within the external locus of control between those dependent on other people (who might follow medical advice) and those who are fatalistic (who may see less reason to comply). Wallston, Wallston, and De Vellis (1978) have distinguished three types of locus of control of relevance to health, internal locus of control, a more fatalistic orientation ('chance'), and reliance on such figures as doctors and other health professionals ('powerful others').

Education

Health care is concerned with education as well as treatment. Relatively low levels of compliance amongst diabetics has been attributed to lack of knowledge about the disease; many patients are aware of this and look to health professionals to learn more. Mason (1985) reports that 27.5 per cent of the diabetics in her sample from a hospital clinic had no idea why tests of urine were necessary, 60 per cent of the patients on tablets perceived a need for more information, and 94.5 per cent of the sample expressed a need for more information about diet. Often it is the principles underlying the information that is lacking. A woman illustrates the confusion that may arise from dietary advice:

> They told me at the hospital to eat plenty of green stuff and all that, and meat, and that's what I do. . . . They tell me not to eat potatoes and somebody else tells me to do the other thing.

When asked what she thought had caused her diabetes she clearly indicated how little she felt she had learnt from her clinic visits:

> Well, she said something about it's something inside here and it attacks us or something.

Many people have advocated formal education programmes. Stone (1961) reported that in a sample of 160 insulin-dependent patients 142 had poor metabolic control. Lack of knowledge was thought to be the main cause in eighty-three cases, four refused to control their diabetes, and fifty-five had social/emotional problems which were thought to explain their poor control. They were studied again after a programme of advice, instruction, and treatment and of the eighty-three originally identified as lacking in information, forty-three later showed good control and four were unwilling to learn. It can be seen therefore that education programmes are not the complete answer to non-compliance. Over a quarter of the original sample remained non-compliant after an education programme.

An additional strategy in tackling non-compliance is needed within the conventional medical consultation to integrate the educational content with a broader psychosocial perspective toward the patient. In the words of Jacobson and Leibovich (1984):

> treatment approaches that emphasise only medical care and information transfer may be less effective than those incorporating psycho-social interventions.

Interventions of this nature are more possible in consultations or therapy sessions in which it is accepted that non-compliance may stem from rational, calculated decisions. The general practitioner is well placed to provide such interventions and opportunistic education is increasingly seen as a vital component of primary care. The major difficulty with achieving this is shortage of time.

Regardless of the setting in which the consultation takes place, the style of communication will influence its effectiveness. Medical descriptions of what is wrong and what the purposes of the treatment regimen are need to be expressed in a way that patients can comprehend. Written explanations to support the consultation may be helpful for patients who simply forget what was said but do not help if the communication is not understood by the patient.

Conclusion

There is a high level of non-compliance amongst diabetics. Some of this results from a lack of knowledge about diabetes and the aims of its treatment; it may be that more effective communication is part of the solution. However, some non-compliance is intentional and the result of patients giving their own meaning to diabetes; they may have other concerns, such as their work, or a general desire to lead a normal life amongst friends, neighbours, and workmates. The recognition of such patterns of thinking in patients involves a more complex psychosocial perspective, that is considering the diabetic in the context of relationships with others.

Chapter five

Diabetics and their social relationships

Introduction

Diabetics live in a social world of family, friends, and other relationships. These relationships may be the source of important practical and emotional help to the diabetic, and may also be a crucial determinant of how an individual adjusts to his or her diabetes. Evidence of the role that social relationships may play as social support for those who are ill is now extensive (Cohen and Syme 1985; Lieberman 1986). The positive aspects of social relationships to diabetics are explored in this chapter. It will also become clear, however, that social and familial ties may not always be beneficial.

The second theme of this chapter is the impact diabetes may have on the individual's relations with others, when its effects extend outwards to affect families and to change wider social relations.

Social relationships and the management of diabetes

Although insulin-dependent diabetics are taught to do their own injections, even as children, they sometimes need help. Sometimes it is a question of a parent or other family member helping with measuring the correct amount of insulin and drawing it up into the syringe. This may also be the case with adult diabetics, either because they are anxious about getting it right, or because they cannot see very well and need someone to check what they are doing. A mother of a 17-year-old diabetic said she still prepared his morning injection:

See where I help him, if he's lazy, I do the morning one, injection, always do, and he does the night one.

Other diabetics are reassured by knowing that someone else in their family knows what to do and would do their injection if necessary. The husband of one diabetic woman not only checked whether she was injecting the correct amount but also said:

If I had to, I would do it for her. I don't say in her stomach, which is where she does it now, but in her arm.

Members of a diabetic's family may also help with monitoring blood sugar levels by checking the results of blood or urine tests. Sometimes it is just a question of confirming what colour the test stick has gone after being dipped into a sample of the patient's urine. The wife of a diabetic said:

He only shows me when it's bright orange, you know. That is the colour, orange, isn't it when it's naughty? He says, 'Look, what have I been eating?'

Some supporters may take the responsibility for doing the analysis of the blood or urine test. One woman in her 70s who lived with her diabetic sister-in-law said:

She has tests three times a day, which I do as she cannot see to do it.

Another practical way in which family members may help diabetics is by making sure that toe-nails are properly cut without the surrounding flesh being cut and infected. Older people may need this help because they cannot see or reach their toe-nails easily and because they have lost some of the sense of feeling in their feet as a result of neuropathy. Children may need to be trained to be particularly careful in cutting their toe-nails.

Diabetics may also receive help in complying with that other important aspect of their treatment regimen, adhering to a diet. Sometimes it is a question of altering the family shopping list so that saccharin replaces sugar, brown bread replaces white, and more fruit and vegetables are bought to provide a diet rich in fibre. Help may also take the form of calculating what exchanges of food can be made while staying within the permitted amount of calories, or making sure that the diabetic person does not eat too much. Sometimes parents, husbands, or wives ensure that a diabetic engaging in anything energetic like playing football, swimming, or dancing has a supply of glucose readily available in case signs of hypo develop. One young diabetic woman had always made sure that:

> Even when we were courting he'd have a packet of glucose in his pocket.

Many husbands and wives become skilled in identifying the signs of an approaching hypo. A diabetic woman said:

> He knows I'm going hypo before I do. He sort of says to me, 'Oy, Glucose' and I say, 'I'm not hypo', but he knows I am even if I don't know. He can tell by my eyes and reactions.

Fletcher, a diabetic doctor (1982: 79), acknowledges such support from his wife:

> In the past twenty years I have become less able to recognize my own hypos and I am deeply grateful to my wife for her help in spotting them.

Apart from giving practical support the families of diabetics may also give social and psychological support which helps in the process of adjusting to the disorder, for example by encouraging the diabetic to see himself or herself as normal and healthy. The spouse or family member is a strong influence in retaining a sense of normality in the context of diabetes. The husband of an elderly diabetic woman was determined not to allow his wife to dwell upon her condition as diabetic:

> I know tons of people who are diabetic . . . but if you start moaning about it, it will get you down. It's a thing you can't help so you pass it off.

This desire by family members to hold on to a sense of normality may sometimes become a case of colluding with the diabetic to normalize behaviour by ignoring some of the constraints required. While this may not be helpful in terms of achieving a satisfactory blood sugar level, it may encourage the sufferer towards a more positive view of the personal meaning of being diabetic. Concern with the diabetic's happiness may weigh more seriously in the spouse's mind than the need to patrol the partner's compliance with diet. As a husband said:

> I don't think it affects her if she does have something to eat that she's not supposed to have because if she likes it and enjoys it, I mean that's half the battle, that's my opinion.

The emotional support provided by a spouse is frequently perceived as the one thing that helps the diabetic to avoid sinking too far into moods of depression. A woman described how her husband helped:

> Sometimes I get depressed. . . . I fly off the handle very quick and I just go berserk, you know. And that is when I think to myself, 'Is it worth it? Why should I bother?' 'What am I doing this for?' And he talks me out of it and I think to myself, 'You're just being silly.'

The family climate can therefore be a useful support to diabetics coping with the practical and psychological problems of adhering to the treatment regimen (Schafer *et al.* 1983; Schlenk and Hart 1984) and in achieving a well-controlled blood sugar level (Edelstein and Linn 1985).

However family environments are not always helpful. In families where there is a lot of conflict, children with diabetes tend to become emotionally involved and their blood sugar levels are affected (Koski and Kumento 1977; Minuchin, Rosman, and Baker 1978). It is now thought likely that many cases of 'brittle' diabetes may be influenced by the increased tension of family quarrels (Lindsay 1985).

Parents and spouses of diabetics are themselves often aware that their role can be harmful as well as beneficial. Attempting to give too much care can be the cause of emotional upsets which may in turn upset the diabetic's blood sugar level. When they insist that diabetics adhere to the treatment regimen exactly as prescribed, they are likely to be seen as being over-protective and rigid. Such attitudes may create family tension and quarrels which are counter-productive in terms of maintaining control of blood sugar levels. Such dilemmas can result in disagreements and indeed conflict between parents as to the amount of help they should give. A young woman described how as a teenager she had been caught between the care of her over-protective father and a mother who bullied her and made no allowance for her diabetes. There were terrible arguments:

> Are you sure you weighed those potatoes properly? It's not a quarter of an ounce over is it? He's very protective. . . . I think he feels guilty, that it's his fault . . . blames himself. I mean I still get regular phone-calls from him [now that she is married].

Her mother, on the other hand, was not very sympathetic:

> I tried to tell my mum about it [a hypo] but she thought I was exaggerating, that I was given to a little crying. My mum never did understand diabetes, she always thought that a hypo was for attention.

Benoliel (1970) examined the different styles that parents may employ to manage the many problems arising from their child's diabetes. In this in-depth study of nine families four styles of parental management were identified. The first style was described as 'protective', where the parent performed most of the diabetic treatment procedures for the child so that they effectively took over decisions about the child's activities. The second style was termed the 'adaptive' style, in which parents progressively encouraged their children to become responsible for diabetic procedures as they grew older. Thirdly, they identified a 'manipulative' style, where parents attempted to get the diabetic procedures carried out by any means that achieved the end, which meant that there was no consistent style of management. This style appeared to be particularly associated with tension arising from endless negotiations between parents and the child. The fourth style was called 'abdicative' and parents who adopted this style played only a minor part in seeing that their child's diabetic procedures and treatment regimen were carried out. Benoliel noted that in only three of the nine families studied did both parents adopt the same style. In the other six families the different styles adopted by parents often seemed to be either the result of existing family conflicts or the cause of new ones. However, five of the nine families did adjust and incorporate the diabetic regimen into 'a way of life'. In the other four families the diabetes of the child continued to be a source of tension and strain which affected the way the child managed the diabetic regimen.

Benoliel argues that the styles of management adopted by parents affect the child not only on a day-to-day basis but also as part of the socialization process in which the child develops an identity and ways of looking at the world:

> the young diabetic's sense of self-esteem is directly related to the emotional climate that is part of his everyday living, and moral judgments about his worth are conveyed mainly through the expressive processes used by his parents.
>
> (Benoliel 1970: 25)

The diabetic child's acceptance of diabetes may also be influenced by brothers and sisters and the extended family of uncles and aunts (Lindsay 1985). A diabetic woman remembered how visiting uncles made her aware of how, as a child, she was different from her brothers and sisters, making it harder for her to accept her diabetic identity:

> My uncles used to call me 'sugar-baby' and I hated it. They did it to comfort me but it didn't. If they had just come round and treated me as one of the kids it would have been different . . . they'd come round and give all the kids a packet of sweets each, but obviously I couldn't have them.

Instead her uncles would give her money but she felt that this too only led to further difficulties; her parents bought her whatever she wanted and this was resented by her brothers and sisters. Such experiences can provide a powerful sense for an individual of being different, and of being disadvantaged because of being different.

People who have become diabetic in adult life may also experience the pressures of over-protective families. In some cases the protective attitudes and behaviour of other family members encourage diabetics to see themselves as sick, rather than being encouraged to adopt a more positive approach. A shopkeeper in his 50s was encouraged by his family to retire and leave the running of the shop to his son and daughter-in-law. He traced his retirement very clearly to their views of him as sick and vulnerable:

> Everybody knows I am diabetic, I shouldn't eat that, I shouldn't eat this. And my son keeps on, 'You must do this'

and that and other things. They feel sympathetic towards me and treat me as a sick person.

This kind of experience may be thought of as socialization into the sick-role. Diabetics are encouraged by family and friends to accept numerous limitations on their lives. The consequences may quite clearly be 'double edged': the individual receives strong reminders about the seriousness of his or her condition and of the importance of adhering to treatment, which may increase some sufferers' ability to comply with the treatment regimen. However such advantages may be at the expense of accepting an unnecessarily cautious, limited, and withdrawn life-style.

Wider social relationships

Wider social relationships with friends and acquaintances play an important part in sustaining the individual's sense of psychological well-being (Cobb 1976), and provide an important sense of support (Carpenter *et al.* 1983). Diabetics who are relatively isolated certainly seem to experience a sense of disadvantage. Social relationships are not necessarily established from mere social contact. A diabetic man who was retired and who lived in a lodging-house found it hard to identify anyone with whom he could talk about his diabetes, despite the fact that he came into contact with large numbers of people:

It's not actual solitude, you see, there are people in the place.

He had only recently been diagnosed and was anxious about how to manage his diabetes. Superficial social relationships arose from occasions where he played cards with others in the lodgings. However numerous concerns in relation to his diabetes could not be discussed with such acquaintances, so he relied very much on visits to the out-patients' clinic at the hospital. Other examples of such extreme social isolation and associated difficulties in adjusting to diabetes were found amongst those attending the same hospital (Kelleher forthcoming). A woman who lived alone and whose diabetes was poorly controlled had no friends that she could identify. If she did not feel well she really had only herself to rely upon: 'I just try to buck myself up.' An important part of her network resources was the community diabetes nurse who called to see her once a week.

Other professions may come to be important influences. School-teachers are an important part of the social network for children, and can be very supportive, for example by being prepared to take diabetic children on school trips. One teenage girl described how she had managed her insulin on a school trip to a holiday camp:

> Well when you get there you just put it in the fridge and go and take it whenever you need it. They were really nice about it.

She conveyed how, especially compared with her parents, the teachers seemed less intrusive and over-protective. But, like parents, some teachers can become over-anxious and try to give too much help. A young woman remembered her teachers on school journeys differently:

> I had no problems but the teachers just wouldn't let go of me. If we went out they were holding my hand . . . and 'Have you eaten, Katherine? You mustn't have that ice-cream' and things like that. They wouldn't treat me as normal, as a normal child. They kept pampering me all the time.

Friendships are a particularly important part of the social network of adolescents and peer group opinions are important in the formation of the diabetic adolescents' views of themselves. Such friendships may help diabetic adolescents to see themselves as normal. One boy, a well-controlled diabetic who played a lot of sport, said:

> I tell all my friends and they treat me the same . . . they ask what it's like, about injections, but that's all really. . . . They just treat me fair.

For others the cost of maintaining their social life requires greater compromises. One teenage girl managed her diet to fit in with her normal social life:

> Well usually I eat something before I go, so when I do go out I don't feel hungry. And if I do go out to a party or anything I won't have anything to eat. I don't usually eat when I go to parties and I don't drink.

Another young woman described the pressures she had experienced as a teenager to join with other teenagers in non-scheduled eating and drinking:

> I used to go up discos and drink, eat a bar of chocolate if I fancied it, eat a bag of crisps . . . then it became, 'Good old Katherine, she's having a good go there tonight, she's having a drink'.

She valued the feeling of being an accepted member of her group, although she acknowledged the penalty that went with full participation in the group, in terms of the fluctuations in her blood sugar level:

> I had nothing but hypos, I was forever dehydrating. I was in hospital for two weeks and then out for two weeks.

Many teenagers with diabetes experience in an extreme form the countervailing pressures experienced by many diabetics, attempting to lead as normal a life as possible with all the associated risks, but restricting many aspects of life to limits which may improve metabolic control and so resulting in a sense of life impoverished or unacceptably different from others.

It is possible to show in a more systematic way how advantages and disruptions in social relationships can be important influences upon the well-being of diabetics. Where studies have attempted to measure objectively the influence of life events such as job changes, evidence has emerged that social changes do have effects upon diabetic control. How such effects occur is less clear. Stress may have a direct influence upon metabolic processes; equally possible is that the disruptive effect of events reduces the care and attention a diabetic can give to maintaining proper dietary and other controls. Life events involving a loss of social relationship can be particularly important in disrupting a diabetic's control of blood sugar level (Hauser and Polletts 1979; Bradley 1979; Revenson 1983). Systematic studies also suggest another interesting possible relationship between social relationships and the course of diabetes, which may be quite different for men and women. A study of thirty-seven non-insulin-dependent diabetics (Heitzman and Kaplan 1984) suggested that men who said that they were very satisfied with their support networks tended to have poorly controlled blood sugar levels, whereas women who said that they were satisfied with their support networks tended to have well-controlled blood sugar levels. One possible interpretation of such findings is that, to the extent that the networks of men and women are different, the friends and other social contacts of men, unlike those of women, are influential in encouraging behaviour that is inappropriate for metabolic control. This would be consistent with other evidence suggesting that male values are responsible for the health problems associated with excessive alcohol consumption or with risky behaviour such as driving cars too fast.

Diabetes and its effects on social relationships

This chapter has considered how social ties may influence the diabetic's well-being; how diabetes affects social relationships is now discussed.

Family life may be influenced in small but significant ways by limitations imposed upon a diabetic from his or her treatment. Family meals may need to be more carefully planned and time-tabled than in non-diabetic families, creating difficulties for whoever takes responsibility for providing meals. Mothers and wives and others who provide food often take pride in giving their children or spouses a large and satisfying meal, but when one of the family is a diabetic this role conception changes. They may become someone with a responsibility for monitoring and controlling the eating of the household or at least someone *expected* to control the eating of the diabetic (Lindsay 1985). This role has, at least initially, far more negative connotations – of monitoring, checking, and denying. An overweight, non-insulin-dependent diabetic described how his wife loved cooking and providing meals for her family. With the onset of his diabetes, however, meal-times became dominated by arguments about what he should or should not be eating. His teenage children would say:

What are you eating that for? What are you doing that for? . . . . What are you giving him that for? She tends to forget that what she gives me sometimes is no good for me.

A diabetic woman said of her husband:

He'll nag me because I don't eat enough and I'm going hypo

. . . and I sort of say to him, 'Don't nag me, it's me that's got it'. . . . But he says, 'It's not you that's got it, it's the family. We've got to cope with it as well as you'.

Another woman described how her diabetic husband had become obsessive about having his meals on time and complained if she was late home from work. He was also worried about the timing of his injections before meals and refused to go out to social occasions.

In some cases the non-diabetic partner attempts to control the diabetic treatment regimen but with results that appear to embitter the whole relationship. One man, through a natural concern for the risks he felt his diabetic wife was undergoing, found himself having to reveal to the hospital specialist the extent of his wife's non-compliance with dietary restrictions. He was compelled to disclose the failings in her diet and felt that there was a sense of betraying his wife as he described the chocolates and sweets she persisted in eating.

Even where such extreme strains in family relationships do not arise, many husbands or wives nevertheless find that they are required to take on an unfamiliar and often difficult role, that of carer. An extreme example of the difficulties created by diabetes was a woman with a diabetic husband whose young son also developed the disorder. With evident bitterness she complained:

I never found living with my husband's diabetes plain sailing and now two diabetics are, at times, exhausting . . .
physically putting the day together around injections, prompt high-fibre meals and dealing with the occasional hypo . . .
can be very distressing for the non-diabetic as well.

(*Balance*, December 1982: 2)

Diabetics can face a number of concerns about forming relationships as they anticipate such difficulties. Some may see themselves as likely to become a burden and an unattractive proposition for a prospective partner. One young man said:

I would make doubly sure that the girl I do go out with or take up with knows the responsibility she would have, because today in this world there are so many responsibilities, so many headaches. . . . I want them to know what they've let themselves in for.

A diabetic may worry about parenting offspring who also prove to be diabetic. This may be perceived as a concern in itself or through anticipating that diabetic children will produce strains on family relationships.

For some men with diabetes, another source of difficulties in forming or sustaining relationships may be sexual problems as a result of impotence. Some women with the disorder may report difficulties with contraception or with a loss of sexual appetite. One insulin-dependent woman said:

> I don't know what it is, it just does not interest me. It's a terrible thing. He's very good [husband] because I mean, on the man, it's very bad for the man, like my husband. It used to cause a lot of arguments at first, but he's come to terms now, he just accepts it.

Diabetes, parenting, and the family

All relationships between parents and children are made up of contrasts of rewarding and frustrating experiences, but the negative aspects may be accentuated if parents are bringing up a diabetic child. Relationships can become strained in a number of ways. A parent may be responsible for giving a young child his or her injections and may therefore be identified in the child's mind with something unpleasant. It is difficult not to be hurt by occasional outbursts such as 'I hate you, Mum' that can easily arise in such circumstances. One particularly frustrating area of child care arises from the inevitable need to discipline children, when it is not always easy to tell whether bad behaviour is caused by an approaching hypo or by intentional misbehaviour on the part of the child. One parent crisply explained:

> It's not always easy to know whether he needs a smack or a sweet.

(Lindsay 1985: 48)

Parents' uncertainty about how to regard bad behaviour may affect the development of the child and cause parents further concern. As children grow older they also grow to be more independent of their parents and the usual struggles about what they may or may not do become further complicated by parents anxious about maintaining the treatment regimen and uncertain of how flexible it can be. Uncertainty about how to respond to the problems presented by a diabetic child may cause or aggravate marital difficulties; the care of a child with a chronic health condition is often associated with significant marital dissension (Lindsay 1985).

Having a diabetic child in the family may affect not only parents but also brothers and sisters, who may feel that the diabetic child gets preferential treatment or is allowed to 'get away with' bad behaviour when they would not. The mother of a diabetic teenager said that her two non-diabetic daughters always complained that

> The girls say I'm all for him, but I'm not. He's not a Mummy's boy. But when there is a row they always bring that up.

A diabetic woman said that she did not get on with her older sister because when they were children her parents had always emphasized to her sister that she should

> Try to agree with Katherine, because you'll upset her diabetes.

Conclusion

This chapter has illustrated the two-way relations between the sufferer of diabetes and his or her social ties. Social relations can influence and shape how the individual experiences diabetes. In turn the effects of the disorder extend outwards to the individual's social world. For many families with a diabetic, none of the problems illustrated in this chapter will prove to be salient or distressing, and it needs to be said that it is easier to convey the difficulties and negative impacts of diabetes on others than it is to express the unremarkable stability of many other diabetic sufferers' social relations.

Chapter six

Issues in the continuing care of diabetics

Introduction

The early diagnosis and initial treatment of diabetes is important, but provision of continuing care for the disorder remains vital. The aims of continuing care provision include monitoring and improving blood sugar levels, screening patients for complications, and educating patients to take greater responsibility for their care. This chapter considers the wide range and diversity of services provided for care, the variety of professions involved, and some of the problems that emerge.

Specialist care

Much of the hospital care provided for diabetics is in the form of special clinics. In some areas of the country there is a shortage of expertise available. A survey conducted in 1983, which covered 234 health districts (97 per cent), revealed that in 30 districts there was no specialist diabetic clinic and in a further 83 districts there was only one specialist clinic. It also appeared that 92 per cent of districts did not have combined clinics with ophthalmologists, 84 per cent did not have educational sessions, 53 per cent did not have a specialist nurse in diabetes, 40 per cent did not have a dark room for retinal examination, 20 per cent did not have a dietician available in the clinic, and 11 per cent did not have any chiropody provision. The report comments that the survey shows 'disturbing evidence of inadequate provision of services' and also notes particularly the 'deficiency in all ophthalmological facilities . . . for up to 80% of blindness due to diabetes may well be preventable' (*Diabetes Update* 1984: 1). A similar conclusion was reached by the Royal College of Physicians (1984: 15) when they conducted a survey of the provision of medical care for adult diabetics. There is also a shortage of facilities for treating the renal problems that diabetics are at risk of developing (National Kidney Research Fund Report 1987). At an international level there is also wide variation in the provision of care available to diabetics (WHO 1985: 67).

Primary care

Despite the deficiencies in the provision of care, the hospital may provide a wide variety of specialist services appropriate to diabetic care. Moreover, some patients think that their diabetes should be managed by hospital doctors whom they see as experts, rather than by GPs who may seem unsure of themselves in dealing with the problems of diabetics. Many simply get their prescriptions from their GP but take their problems to the specialist in the hospital. One diabetic said of her GP:

Mention the word diabetic and he comes out in a sweat. . . .
I can go to him for dressings for my leg, but that's about all.

None the less in view of the current limitations of specialist services much of the responsibility for diabetic care falls to primary care. There are some GPs who are keen to take on the continuing care of diabetics and a number of successful schemes have been set up, often in conjunction with hospital specialists (Hill 1979; Thorn and Russell 1973; Williams 1985). There are several advantages in the continuing care being with GPs. First, diabetes is a common complaint and the average GP list will include approximately thirty diabetic patients, so GPs should learn about diabetic care. Second, diabetes affects other body systems and is affected by the family and the social situation of the diabetic person, and is exactly the kind of health problem that GPs are well suited to deal with. GPs usually know more about the family situation of the diabetic than hospital doctors. Patients are also likely to find visits to their GP less time consuming than visits to a crowded out-patient clinic.

In terms of controlling patients' blood sugar levels the schemes are as successful as the hospital out-patient clinics (Porter 1979;

Yudkin, Boucher, and Schopfein 1980; Baksi *et al.* 1984). They are also preferred by many patients (Baksi *et al.* 1984). One patient in such a scheme said approvingly:

> They call me once every three months; they do it at the surgery . . . which saves time. . . . Once a twelve month you go to the surgery for a complete check through, right the way through, needles in the feet, blood test, heart beat, everything. You get the lot.

Studies of GP care in districts where special schemes have not been set up and where GPs have not been given additional support present a less satisfactory picture (Hayes and Harris 1984; Jarrett 1986). A survey of GP care in one English county showed some worrying gaps in the care provided (Mellor *et al.* 1985); 53 per cent reported that they never checked the visual acuity of their diabetic patients. This suggests that retinopathy would not be recognized and treated. Over 40 per cent felt that they did not have sufficient time for the routine care of diabetics. A particularly revealing observation from the study was that the majority of GPs preferred their patients' urine not to be entirely free of sugar; they may share patients' concerns of the need to avoid hypoglycaemic attacks. Nevertheless it was encouraging that 80 per cent expressed interest in terms of a willingness to attend post-graduate courses if provided.

The division of labour

Apart from the hospital doctors, their laboratory support staff, and GPs working in the primary care sector, there is a range of other health care professionals who can contribute to the continuing care of diabetics. Dieticians and chiropodists have a recognized role in continuing care, as do ophthalmologists, but in some clinics, paediatricians, specialist diabetic nurses, health visitors, psychologists, and psychiatrists may also be involved.

At least two fundamental issues of policy are unresolved in diabetic care. First, who should take primary responsibility, the hospital or the GP? Second, to what extent diabetic care can be performed by specialist nurses. Day (1987: 21) states:

> We analysed our clinic and at least half of the diabetics

attending do not need a medical examination. Most have come for counselling in diabetic control and the specialist nurse is ideal to do this.

In another district the community diabetic nurse also took diabetic clinics at a GP's surgery. She suggested that diabetics might be more honest in talking to nurses about their eating habits and blood sugar level monitoring than they would be with a doctor. Some argue that health visitors could play a bigger role in the community care of diabetics (Richards 1983). A recent survey in Leicestershire (Mellor *et al.* 1985) found that all GPs saw health visitors as a resource useful in the care of diabetics, often providing dietary advice.

The issue of who should be centrally concerned in the care of diabetics comes more sharply into focus in the work of education and counselling.

Education

The need for continuing education of diabetics and their families has long been recognized, and many programmes for improving diabetics' knowledge of diabetes have been developed. These range from the one-to-one exchange between doctor and patient to formal education programmes with groups of patients. Regardless of context, these have usually concentrated on the technical and medical aspects of diabetes rather than on psychosocial matters and the assumption is that as the patients learn more about their illness so they will be able to improve their control.

While some aspects of education do take place in the process of medical consultation more formal education groups have been established in most countries. The European Diabetes Education Study Group was established in 1979 and an education section of the British Diabetic Association in 1983. There are also Diabetic Education Associations in the USA, Canada, and Australia. In addition local support groups for diabetics have been established with the guidance of national associations which often provide educational opportunities. These meetings provide an opportunity for people to ask questions about technological developments such as new ways of delivering insulin, new kinds of tablets or insulin, and improvement in the monitoring of blood sugar levels.

Many argue that the education programmes should not only be directed to patients but also aim to inform doctors and the general public about how diabetes affects people in their day-to-day lives, which might lessen the stigmatization of diabetics in the areas of employment, insurance, and the forming of personal relationships.

Research studies on the effect of education programmes on diabetics' adherence or control have shown that didactic programmes have little impact (Fisher *et al.* 1982), which raises questions about the structure, content, and goals of these programmes. Jarrett (1986) comments that many of those treating diabetics have become aware that many education programmes have been neither systematic nor very successful and their expectations may be too high. Education programmes attempt to impose changes in life-style which patients are frequently unwilling or unable to accept, and changes in medical advice as the understanding of diabetes develops cause difficulties for the diabetic who has previously learned other forms of management, particularly in the area of diet.

Historically dietary recommendations have varied enormously, even to the extent of advising a high sugar intake (Bliss 1983). More recently the diet recommended for European and American diabetics has been based on the principle of reducing the carbohydrate content of the diet as carbohydrate foods supply a quickly available source of glucose. This diet was not however based on firm experimental evidence:

> Many of the traditional beliefs concerning the diabetic diet are
> unproven and some may be wrong. Scientific investigation
> has contributed less than it should to dietary theory and
> practice.
>
> (British Diabetic Association 1983: 1)

There has been a gradual realization that a dietary policy based on a low intake of carbohydrates tended to produce a diet which was high in fat content, thus increasing the risk of heart disease, and was therefore not to be recommended to diabetics. In 1979 the American Diabetic Association recommended a high-fibre diet, where what was important was the total energy value rather than the carbohydrate content. The British Diabetic Association followed suit in 1983; this represented a sudden change to an essential part of treatment requiring considerable adjustment by diabetics.

Compliance with dietary recommendations is notoriously poor (Thomas 1981; Jarrett 1986) and the new diet may not be any more successful as a therapy. Several issues seem likely to be involved in this poor compliance, creating a difficult problem for any education programme which attempts to achieve behaviour change. While there is agreement about the importance of controlling the food intake of diabetics, the scientific basis on which the recommended diet is based is not well enough grounded, and some doctors convey only generalized dietary advice to patients. This may be the result of the doctors' own limited knowledge of dietary principles (West 1973) or the fact that doctors may not have sufficient knowledge of the work patterns and life-styles of their patients to be able to recommend an appropriate diet for individual patients (West 1973; Nuttall 1983). Furthermore dietary advice may not be followed because the professionals treating diabetics see food as a problem and fail to consider the social and emotional functions of eating. The patient and the patient's family are likely to see food and meals not only as an exercise in nutrition (Hinkle 1962), but also as social activities which fulfil a range of social and emotional functions. Attempts to control a person's eating may therefore be a much more invasive therapy than is realized.

The problems of incorporating the contents of education programmes into a diabetic's life have led to an increased application of patient-centred education where the patient is an active participant in decisions rather than a passive recipient of information. The WHO report contrasts this approach with traditional medical practice:

> Traditional medical practice is based on diagnosis and cure of pathological conditions, with the patient playing a passive role. . . . In contrast, patient education in the treatment of chronic illness . . . requires the active participation of the patient.
>
> (WHO 1985: 81)

Counselling and other psychological interventions

Diabetes can bring with it a range of personal problems for the diabetic individual and the family. While continuing education programmes for diabetics are likely to improve the management of the disease, most do not tackle these social-psychological problems. Counselling has been developed to cope with these issues which may range from interpersonal and psychological problems, such as sexual impotence, through to coping with housing which is limiting the mobility of a diabetic person with poor eyesight or an amputation. A diabetic man said that he felt in need of counselling because

> I have been a single parent for the past ten years and during these years have shielded the children [aged 13, 19, 21] from problems and troubles including my diabetes as I feel the children, with all the additional problems of being a single parent family, have enough already.
>
> (*Balance* 1984: 16)

One function of counselling is to give patients an opportunity to air their feelings and concerns which may not be possible in the home environment. This is illustrated by one man:

> I felt I was alone with my problems. I couldn't burden my wife with worries. . . . I saw only my limitations wherever I looked. . . . I felt despair and an inner revolt.
>
> (Gfeller and Assal 1983)

Several different versions of group and individual counselling have been tried out but few have been evaluated. Gfeller and Assal (1983: 208–9) report the results of their programme which involved weekly 'Round Table Discussions', 'which include fifteen to twenty patients and other people significant in the patients' lives [and] last for one and a half hours. All patients as well as physicians, nurses and dieticians of the Unit have to participate'. They argue that these sessions provide 'a good atmosphere for patients to verbalise emotions . . . while also allowing the medical team to discover the patients' subjective experiences'. The sessions are said to be very instructive for the professionals who are mostly engaged in listening to the accounts of patients.

There is obviously a range of ways of providing diabetics with counselling to help them cope with the varied problems they may encounter in their attempts to manage their roles and the expectations others have of them. Most of the ways tried so far seem to aim to provide an outlet for patients' feelings and to give doctors knowledge of these feelings, but pay little attention to providing constructive help about either relationships or problems connected with work and employment. There have been some notable exceptions which have attempted to broaden the range of issues to be tackled. These approaches may be more aptly described as forms of psychotherapy.

Groen and Pelser reported on a series of group therapy sessions they organized over a period of eighteen months involving thirty-five patients. Although they say that as they had no control group they were unable to determine whether their patients were better controlled in terms of blood sugar level at the end of the experimental period, the patients were unanimous that the group approach was of great value for their emotional support (Groen and Pelser 1982: 177). The problems discussed were both 'technical' and 'life' problems; many life problems concerned ambivalent relationships between the patients and their parents (in the young patients, especially mothers), marriage partners, and the treating physicians. The physicians were felt to be mainly interested in their urine and blood sugar levels and were not seen to have time to discuss the difficulties of having to live with diabetes (Groen and Pelser 1982: 175). The impact of psychotherapy on both metabolic control and psychological adjustment has been a recent subject of some well-controlled studies (Sonksen, Ryle, and Milton 1987).

At the moment doctors, nurses, or other professionals may take on a counselling role because they are there when the help is needed or because they enjoy that aspect of the work, but they may have had no training in counselling and have no knowledge of other resources they could call on. A recent conference report of the BDA emphasizes the difficulties that counselling may create for the members of the medical team:

> Counselling is an unnatural skill for team members – it
> embraces many unfamiliar techniques and involves
> interaction both up and down the social scale. Staff will be

taken out of their traditional roles and not all will be prepared to carry it out.

(British Diabetic Association 1987: 9)

Kantrow (1963) has advocated that special diabetic counsellors should be employed; while yet another professional becoming involved in the care and treatment of diabetics might only complicate matters, the community diabetic nurses could take on this role once they had received appropriate counselling training.

Stress and its management have been another area where psychological treatments have been usefully applied. A considerable amount of research shows that stress does affect blood sugar levels, although some writers are critical of the methods of this research (Fisher *et al.* 1982; Barglow *et al.* 1984; Bradley 1985). Relaxation techniques are strongly advocated to reduce stress levels and improve metabolic control (Fitzgerald 1984). Hodgkinson goes as far as saying that

I believe the role of diet as a means of controlling the diabetic condition has been exaggerated. Over emphasis of this aspect of the diabetic life has contributed to the neglect of what I am sure is the crucial role played by the mind-body mechanisms.

(Hodgkinson 1984: 138)

Other writers are more cautious (Fisher *et al.* 1982) but many see the possibilities in using relaxation techniques and argue that more research needs to be conducted to identify those individuals where it might successful (Bradley 1985).

Costs

The final issue in the continuing care and treatment of diabetes is the cost involved to both the individual and the state. The costs of medication and diet may impose significant financial hardship on the individual diabetic. In some countries there may be some state assistance. For example in the UK diabetics receive their insulin and tablets on prescription and are exempt from prescription charges. Some may be eligible for an addition to their supplementary pension towards the cost of food, but most receive no help towards the cost of paying for a healthy diet or for special diabetic foods and drinks. Until 1987 most diabetics also had to buy the more convenient disposable syringes. They still have to buy the equipment for monitoring their own blood sugar level if they prefer to measure their blood directly rather than use the less accurate method which requires them to put a dipstick into a sample of their urine. Diabetics may also suffer financial costs as a result of their condition being viewed unfavourably by employers and insurance companies.

Many diabetics face restrictions in the area of work they may undertake. They frequently need advice as to why they will not be accepted for, or may have to give up, work involving driving heavy goods vehicles or using heavy machinery. Jobs which involve frequent changes of shifts are also unsuitable for diabetics as they upset the pattern of meals and injections. These restrictions limit the areas of paid employment open to diabetics (Petrides 1981). The BDA has recently commissioned a study to examine the difficulties experienced by diabetics in finding suitable employment (Robinson 1987). Some diabetics feel that they are being unfairly discriminated against when they are refused jobs for which they are suitable. In a survey of 366 diabetics in Glasgow 6 per cent said that they had been refused work because of their diabetes (Hutchinson, Kesson, and Slater 1983). An earlier study (Kantrow 1963) showed that 53 per cent of insulin-dependent diabetics said that they had been refused work because of their diabetes. One young insulin-dependent man who wanted to be an ambulance driver understood why that was not possible but said:

But I think it does stop you in other areas. I've applied for quite a few jobs but I get turned down. I've never known why.

Diabetics are eligible to register as disabled, but while this could help in gaining employment, many diabetics fail to register largely because they wish to avoid the stigma they feel is attached to the label 'disabled' (British Diabetic Association 1983).

The costs of state provision vary widely according to the organization of public and private health care. In the UK the costs through the National Health Service of treating diabetes is considerable. In the year 1979/80 the cost of diabetic treatment was 1 per cent of the annual National Health Service revenue and the total cost to the state was estimated to be £161.3m (Jarrett

1986). The level of service resulting from this financial provision is none the less recognized as being inadequate (*Diabetes Update* 1984; Royal College of Physicians 1984; National Kidney Research Fund Report 1987).

Conclusion

In the continuing care and treatment of diabetic people, there are debates concerning the kind of education and counselling that should be provided, and whether the care should be in the hands of GPs working in the primary sector of health care or hospital specialists. The question of the role of stress and how it can be managed are areas where further research is needed. Diabetic treatment imposes a considerable financial burden on both the individual and the state.

Chapter seven

Prospects and overview

Most of the recent developments and current research in diabetes are concerned with controlling the central diagnostic criterion of diabetes, a raised level of blood sugar. If blood sugar levels can be well controlled not only can the symptoms be eliminated but also the onset of life-threatening complications can be postponed or avoided altogether.

The main line of research has been the search for better ways of delivering insulin to where it is needed in the body. The discovery of insulin in 1922 was, of course, a major development which has increased the life-span of many people, but injecting into an arm or leg two or three times a day is a very crude and unnatural way of replacing insulin. Much research has therefore tried to find ways of delivering insulin which are physiologically more similar to the way it is supplied naturally in non-diabetic people.

It has been recognized that improvements could be made to the system which stabilizes an insulin-dependent diabetic on a daily amount of insulin to be injected before meals but in any one of a number of sites on the body. Insulin injected into a thigh, for example, is likely to be less quickly available than insulin injected into the stomach (Berger 1985). Recently it has been suggested that long-acting insulin should form a smaller proportion of the daily insulin dose and that diabetics themselves should boost their basal insulin by an injection of short-acting insulin just before meals and according to what they need (Berger 1985).

Technological developments have facilitated these new emphases in the delivery of insulin. The aim has been to produce a mechanism which could be implanted into the body and which would monitor the level of sugar in the blood and supply insulin as necessary. Such a mechanism would be like that part of the pancreas which supplies insulin in non-diabetics. Some progress has been made towards developing such a closed-loop system but not all of the technical problems have yet been overcome (Schade and Eaton 1985).

Now available are battery-powered pumps which are strapped on to the body and are connected to a needle inserted into the stomach. These continuous subcutaneous insulin infusion (CSII) pumps supply a continuous trickle of insulin into the body, and are fitted with a control which allows the wearer to give a variable booster amount of insulin prior to a meal. The amount of insulin administered has to be calculated by the doctor and then, on a day-to-day basis, by the diabetic rather than by the natural balancing processes of the endocrine system. This system of supplying insulin (an open-loop system) therefore requires the diabetic person to monitor their blood sugar level carefully and regularly and to replenish the supply of insulin in the pump.

The infusion pumps can help to achieve better glycaemic control, but whether this is achieved depends on the willingness and ability of the individual to do the necessary monitoring (Dupre 1985; Ward 1986). Not all insulin-dependent diabetics are suitable patients to be fitted with pumps. There are also greater risks of localized infections and of ketoacidosis occurring (Pickup et al. 1985). This problem involves a serious lack of insulin causing the body to use up body fats and producing ketones in the urine, drowsiness, and vomiting. Episodes of ketoacidosis may be associated with stress brought on by either infection or emotional upsets. Infusion pumps are also expensive, costing in the region of £500–£1,500 (Ward 1986).

The reactions of diabetic people using pumps has generally been favourable (Pickup et al. 1985). The combination of the background trickle of insulin being continuously supplied by the pump and the facility for giving a booster just before a meal does give greater flexibility to people, allowing them to delay meals for an hour or so without worrying, and generally improving their quality of life. However, as Bradley (1987) notes, few treatments are evaluated in terms of their effect on the quality of life, although they should be. Some diabetics do find the pump intrusive and inhibiting in some physical activities although it can be unplugged for short periods, when taking a bath for example. Some feel less in control of their diabetes when they have an electromechanical pump strapped to them, and there is the risk that people wearing a visible pump will be stigmatized (Pollans and Turkat 1984).

Implantable insulin pumps which are in the process of development would not be visible, but those tried so far have a number of other disadvantages (Home 1984; Schade and Eaton 1985). There are problems in refilling the pump and of not being able to adjust the rate at which insulin is administered once the pump has been implanted. At present conventional injections are necessary at meal times, but improved technology may soon allow changes in the rate to be made through an external control unit.

A further development is the construction of an 'artificial pancreas' which registers the level of blood glucose and supplies the amount of insulin needed to maintain a normal level of blood glucose. The machines currently in operation are rather large and complex and not suitable for implantation, but can be used for diabetic patients in intensive care. Before an implantable artificial pancreas can be developed it will be necessary to develop a reliable and accurate sensor of blood sugar level which can be linked to a pump.

An alternative to technological approaches is the use of transplants; the first transplant of a pancreas was in 1966 (Sutherland et al. 1985; Hu Yuan-feng et al. 1985). Although pancreas transplants, whether of the whole pancreas or just the islets of Langerhan part, experience the usual risk of being rejected, eventually pancreas transplants could become as frequent and successful as kidney transplants.

Research studies to find better ways of delivering insulin into the body have explored the possibility of packaging insulin doses in a form which would protect insulin from the action of other enzymes until it arrived in the liver. Ideally the packaging would then release the insulin for use, which would overcome the problem of injecting and so improve the quality of life of diabetics, but would not eliminate the need for monitoring blood sugar levels. Attempts have also been made to deliver insulin through the nose but this has not seemed a promising development (Berger 1985).

One recent and successful development in the treatment of

diabetes has been the introduction of human insulin. Although the production of human insulin is a triumph of biotechnology, the insulin itself is not thought to have much in the way of clinical advantages over the existing bovine or porcine insulin (Berger 1985). However its production is likely to bring huge commercial benefits to those companies involved (Erlichman 1982).

Apart from attempts to improve the treatment of diabetes, research is also going on to attempt to identify the causal mechanisms of diabetes and any viral agents which may be involved.

Perhaps what is lacking in diabetes research is sufficient attention to projects which would improve the quality of life of diabetics, particularly the majority of diabetics who are treated by diet and tablets. The difficulties they describe are real problems which require attention if existing treatments are ever going to be successfully applied in the everyday world.

Summary

Chapter 1 outlined the types of diabetes and the nature of the disease syndrome. The classification of diabetes has changed as many cases did not easily fit into the older typologies of maturity onset and juvenile onset or Type I and Type II. The present typology (recommended by WHO 1985) IDDM and NIDDM is not completely satisfactory either, being based on the type of treatment prescribed rather than on clearly defined aetiological differences. The aetiological mechanisms of diabetes have been briefly outlined and the contribution of epidemiological and genetic evidence to understanding has been recognized. The epidemiological evidence relating diabetes to differences of sex, class, and ethnic background were described but not found significant as a general feature of research studies. It was suggested that there is some evidence of an increased incidence of IDDM in the UK and an increased incidence of NIDDM in most parts of the world, particularly in populations where changes to a more industrial society produced greater affluence and a more sedentary lifestyle. However such evidence is insufficient to contribute clear ideas about the causes of diabetes.

Chapter 2 described how individuals experience diabetes. Reactions to the diagnosis and individuals' accounts of their continuing symptoms of tiredness, irritability, loss of feeling, and poor eyesight were described. Diabetics' fears of complications, of their children developing diabetes, and of hypos were also explored. It is these negative aspects of diabetics' lives that are more salient when trying to piece together the experience of the disorder; however for many individuals and for much of the time such problems are not so prominent.

Chapter 3 illustrated how the treatment regimen is an important part of the experience of diabetes. For many people living with diabetes is a matter of balancing the experience of symptoms and the fear of complications against the scheduling of life and the regulation of eating that treatment regimens require. Treatment regimens which involve control of eating, scheduled meals, and monitoring of urine or blood sugar level impose a pattern on the life-style of diabetics which reduces the possibilities for spontaneous, unplanned social activities. For teenagers these constraints make their normal attempts to achieve a measure of independence difficult for both them and their parents. Many diabetics find the task of selecting what they can eat by consulting a list of 'exchanges' too complicated and settle instead for eating a limited range of food for many years. Some people view their diabetes entirely in terms of its practical problems and challenges, which tends to result in a distinctive way of coping with the disorder. Other people may see their diabetes as something which not only presents them with problems but also disrupts their normal sense of self; such perceptions require the individual to cope by somehow reducing the significance of their disorder. Strategies were examined such as minimizing the significance of symptoms and avoiding those social situations where they feel their identity as a normal person might be vulnerable. There are times though when diabetes is seen neither as a series of practical problems nor as a threat to a normal identity which can be managed. At such times moods of depression are commonly experienced.

Discussing the practical and psychological problems posed by the treatment regimens led in Chapter 4 to an examination of the widespread non-adherence to treatment. Adherence means more than taking injections or tablets. Keeping to a diet demands changes in behaviour, which may challenge long-established preferences and cultural beliefs and may also affect other members of a diabetic's family or social network. The extent of non-compliance and correlation of the behaviour with other variables such as educational level were briefly discussed. Such basic characteristics do not usually provide sufficient explanations for non-compliance. After examining diabetics' accounts, the intentions of such actions need to be considered more closely. Individuals weigh up the costs of complying with particular aspects of the treatment regimen, for example monitoring blood sugar levels or keeping to a diet, against the benefits of reduced risks of long-term complications. This balancing is done by reference to their own beliefs about health and by weighing the values they attach to their present life-style and social relations. Lack of knowledge about diabetes also contributes to non-compliance and greater emphasis should be given to improving the communication of information in health care. In particular information that is relevant to the personal concerns of the individual may well enhance adherence.

Chapter 5 described the effects of social relationships on diabetes. The family can be a major influence on diabetics, by giving both practical and psychological support. Sometimes family relationships can be seen as too protective however, and this may cause conflict. Tensions in family relationships are likely to have an adverse effect on diabetics' control of their blood sugar levels. Diabetes may also affect social relationships as well as being affected by them. The roles of people in the family may alter and the diabetic's social network may also become restricted.

Chapter 6 examined the roles of professionals involved in the care and treatment of diabetics. Education and counselling facilities and the management of stress were discussed. Difficulties in finding suitable employment and the general costs both to the individual and to the state were described.

Conclusion

The description of the day-to-day experience of diabetes makes clear that it affects the lives of people in a whole range of ways. The treatment regimen imposes a pattern on the lives of diabetics which controls their use of time and reduces spontaneity in social life. For many people, their diabetes not only requires a change of behaviour, but also changes their view of themselves.

Given the demands of the treatment and the fact that it is largely concerned with preventing complications in the distant future, it is not so remarkable that many diabetics choose not to comply with all aspects of the treatment. Although providing better education about diabetes may reduce some non-compliance, it will not reduce that which is the result of a weighing-up of priorities rather than a result of ignorance.

The treatment of diabetes is not concerned only with measuring blood sugar levels. An attempt must be made to consider what effects diabetes and the treatment regimen are having on an individual's life. Good care has to be directed towards restoring a diabetic person to an active and satisfying life as well as achieving a better metabolic balance. The personal concerns of the diabetic patient and of the family increasingly need to be brought to the fore in the provision of health care.

References

Alogna, M. (1980) 'Perception of severity of disease and health locus of control in compliant and non-compliant diabetic patients', *Diabetes Care* 3 (4): 533–4.

Aveline, M., McCulloch, D., and Tattersall, R. (1985) 'The practice of group psychotherapy with adult insulin-dependent diabetics', *Diabetic Medicine* 2: 275–82.

Baksi, A., Brand, J., Nicholas, M., Tavabie, A., Cartwright, B., and Waterfield, M. (1984) 'Non-consultant peripheral clinics: a new approach to diabetic care', *Health Trends* 16: 38–40.

Balance (1982) 'Your hypos – you tell us about them', London: British Diabetic Association, October.

Balance (1983) Experts' replies to readers' letters, London: British Diabetic Association, December.

Balance (1984) 'Diabetic after-care: you reply', London: British Diabetic Association, April.

Balance (1985) Letters, 'Perfect diabetic', London: British Diabetic Association, June: 2.

Barglow, P., Hatcher, R., Edidin, D., and Sloan-Rossiter, D. (1984) 'Stress and metabolic control in diabetes: psychosomatic evidence and evaluation of methods', *Psychosomatic Medicine* 46 (2): 127–44.

Barker, D., Gardner, M., and Power, C. (1982) 'Incidence of diabetes amongst people aged 18–50 years in nine British towns: a collaborative study', *Diabetologia* 22: 421–5.

Becker, M. (1974) (ed.) 'The health belief model and personal health behavior', *Health Education Monographs* 2: 324–73.

Becker, M. and Maiman, L. (1980) 'Strategies for enhancing patient compliance', *Journal of Community Health* 6 (2): 113–35.

Benedek, T. (1948) 'An approach to the study of the diabetic', *Psychosomatic Medicine* 10: 248–7.

Bennett, P. H. (1983) 'Diabetes in developing countries and unusual populations', in J. Mann, K. Pyorala, and A. Teuscher (eds) *Diabetes in Epidemiological Perspective*, London: Churchill Livingstone.

Benoliel, J. (1970) 'The developing diabetic identity: a study of family influence', *Community Nursing Research* 3: 14–32.

Berger, M. (1985) Insulin therapy: conventional, in K. Alberti and L. Krall (eds) *The Diabetes Annual 1*, Amsterdam: Elsevier Science Publications.

Bliss, M. (1983) *The Discovery of Insulin*, Edinburgh: Harris.

Bodansky, H. (1986) 'Tales from the diabetic clinic', *Practical Diabetes* 3 (5): 247–8.

Bradley, C. (1979) 'Life events and the control of diabetes mellitus', *Journal of Psychosomatic Research* 23: 159–62.

Bradley, C. (1985) 'Psychological aspects of diabetes', in K. Alberti and L. Krall (eds) *The Diabetes Annual 1*, Amsterdam: Elsevier Science Publications.

Bradley, C. (1987) 'People and pumps', *Balance* 98: 12–15, London: British Diabetic Association.

Bradley, C., Brewin, C., Gamsu, D., and Moses, J. (1984) 'Development of scales to measure perceived control of diabetes mellitus and diabetes related health beliefs', *Diabetic Medicine* 1: 213.

British Diabetic Association (1983) 'Dietary recommendations for diabetics for the 1980s – a policy statement', London: British Diabetic Association.

British Diabetic Association (1987) *Reports from Workshops*, third annual conference, Education Section Group A, London: British Diabetic Association.

Brownlee-Duffeck, M., Peterson, L., Simonds, J., Kilo, C., Goldstein, D., and Hoette, S. (1987) 'The role of health beliefs in the regimen adherence and metabolic control of adolescents and adults with diabetes mellitus', *Journal of Consulting and Clinical Psychology* 55 (2): 139–44.

Campbell, I. and McCulloch, D. (1979) 'Marital problems of diabetics', *Practitioner* (222): 343–56, March.

Carpenter, B., Hansson, R., Rowntree, R., and Jones, W. H. (1983) 'Relational competence and adjustment in diabetic patients', *Journal of Social and Clinical Psychology* 1 (4): 359–69.

Cerkoney, K. and Hart, L. (1980) 'The relationship between the health belief model and compliance of persons with diabetes mellitus', *Diabetes Care* 3 (5): 594–8.

Clements, R. (1986) 'New therapies for the chronic complications of older patients', *American Journal of Medicine* 80 (suppl. 5A).

Cobb, S. (1976) 'Social support as a moderator of life-stress', *Psychosomatic Medicine* 38 (5): 300–14.

S. Cohen, and S. L. Syme, (eds) (1985) *Social Support and Health*, London: Academic Press.

Davis, F. (1961) 'Deviance disavowal: the management of strained interaction by the visibly handicapped', in W. Filstead (ed.) (1972) *An Introduction to Deviance: Readings in the Process of Making Deviants*, Chicago, Ill: Rand McNally.

Davis, F. (1963) *Passage through Crisis: Polio Victims and their Families*, Indianapolis, Ind: Bobbs-Merrill.

Day, D. (1987) 'Not the diabetic clinic', *Balance* Feb/March: 20–1, London: British Diabetic Association.

Diabetes Update (1983) 'Diabetes and driving', London: British Diabetic Association, May: 1.

Diabetes Update (1984) 'Provision of diabetic care in the UK – how good is it?', London: British Diabetic Association, December.

Drummond, N. (1985) 'Against doctors' orders', *New Society* 4 October.

Dunn, S. and Turtle, J. (1981) 'The myth of the diabetic personality', *Diabetes Care* 4 (6): 640–6.

Dupre, J. (1985) 'Open-loop continuous insulin infusion in the management of insulin requiring diabetes mellitus', in K. Alberti and L. Krall (eds) *The Diabetes Annual 1*, Amsterdam: Elsevier Science Publications.

Durranty, P., Ruiz, F., and Garcia de la Rios, M. (1979) 'Age at diagnosis and seasonal variations in the onset of insulin dependent diabetes mellitus in Chile', *Diabetologia* 17: 357–60.

Edelstein, J. and Linn, M. (1985) 'The influence of the family on control of diabetes', *Social Science and Medicine* 21 (5): 541–4.

Employment (DH 131) (1983) London: British Diabetic Association.

Erlichman, J. (1982) 'Biochemists go to war – and UK is battleground', *Guardian* 15 September: 13.

Fisher, E. Delameter, A., Bertelson, A., and Kirkley, B. (1982) 'Psychological factors in diabetes and its treatment', *Journal of Consulting and Clinical Psychology* 50 (6): 993–1,003.

FitzGerald, L. (1984) 'Yoga and diabetes', *Balance* 83 October.

Fletcher, C. (1982) 'Avoiding diabetic disabilities without loss of freedom', *Journal of Royal College of Physicians* 16 (2): 78–9.

Folkman, S. and Lazarus, R. (1980) 'An analysis of coping in a middle-aged community sample', *Journal of Health and Social Behaviour* 21: 219–39.

Fris, R. and Nanjundappa, G. (1986) 'Diabetes, depression and employment status', *Social Science and Medicine* 23 (5) : 471–5.

Fuller, J. (1983) 'Diabetes mortality: a new light on an underestimated public health problem', *Diabetologia* 24: 336–41.

Gabriele, A. J. and Marble, A. (1949) 'Experiences with 116 juvenile campers in a new summer camp for diabetic boys', *American Journal of Medical Science* 218: 161–71.

Gfeller, R. and Assal, J.-Ph. (1983) 'Developmental stages of patient acceptance in diabetes', *Diabetes Education* (2nd European Symposium): 207–18.

Gill, G., Husband, D., Walford, S., Marshall, S., Home, P., and Alberti, K. (1985) 'Clinical feature of brittle diabetes – the Newcastle experience', in J. Pickup (ed.) *Brittle Diabetes*, Oxford: Blackwell Scientific Publications.

Goldgewicht, C., Slema, G., Papoz, L., and Tchobroutsky, G. (1983)

'Hypoglycaemic reactions in 172 type 1(insulin-dependent) diabetic patients', *Diabetologia* 24: 95–9.

Graber, A. L., Christman, Alogna, M., and Davidson, J. (1977) 'Evaluation of diabetes patient education programs', *Diabetes* 26 (1): 61–4.

Greene D. (1986) 'Acute and chronic complications of diabetes mellitus in older patients', *American Journal of Medicine* 80 (suppl. 5A) 39–53.

Groen, J. and Pelser, H. (1982) 'Psycho-social aspects in the therapy of diabetes', *Paediatric and Adolescent Endocrinology* 10: 168–77.

Haber, L. and Smith, R. (1971) 'Disability and deviance: normative adaptation of role behaviour', *American Sociological Review* 36: 87–97.

Hamman, R. (1983) 'Diabetes in affluent societies', in J. Mann, K. Pyorala, and A. Teuscher (eds) *Diabetes in Epidemiological Perspective*, London: Churchill Livingstone.

Hauser, S. and Polletts, D. (1979) 'Psychological aspects of diabetes mellitus: a critical review', *Diabetes Care* 2 (2): 227–32.

Hayes, T. and Harris, J. (1984) 'Randomized controlled trial of routine general practice care for type 2 diabetics', *British Medical Journal* 289: 728–30.

Heitzman, C. and Kaplan, R. (1984) 'Interaction between sex and social support in the control of type 2 diabetes mellitus', *Journal of Consulting and Clinical Psychology*, 52 (6): 1,087–89.

Helgason, T. and Jonasson, M. (1981) 'Evidence for a food additive as a cause of ketosis-prone diabetes', *Lancet* 2: 716–20.

Hill, R. D. (1979) 'Managing the diabetic patient in general practice', *Modern Medicine* July: 56–63.

Hinkle, L. (1962) 'Customs, emotions, and behavior in the dietary treatment of diabetes', *Journal of the American Dietetic Association* 41: 341–4.

Hodgkinson, N. (1984) *Will to be Well*, London: Hutchinson.

Home, P. (1984) 'Implantable insulin infusion pumps', *Balance* 84: 9–11, London: British Diabetic Association.

Hopper, S. (1981) 'Diabetes as a stigmatized condition: the case of lower income clinic patients', *Social Science and Medicine* 15b: 11–19.

Hu Yuan-feng, Zhang Hong, Zang Hong-de, Shao An-hua, LiLi-xian, Zhou Hui-quing, Zao Bao-hua, Zhou Yu-gu, (1985) 'Culture of human fetal pancreas and islet transplantion in 24 patients with type 1 diabetes mellitus', *Chinese Medical Journal* 98(4): 236–43.

Hulka, B., Cassel, J., Kupper, L., and Burdette, J. (1976) 'Communication, compliance and concordance between physicians and patients with prescribed medications', *American Journal of Public Health* 66: 847–53.

Hutchinson, S., Kesson, C., and Slater, S. (1983) 'Does diabetes affect employment prospects?' *British Medical Journal* 287: 946–7.

Jacobson, A. and Leibovich, J. (1984) 'Psychological issues in diabetes mellitus', *Psychosomatics* 25: 7–15.

Jarrett, R. J. (1986) *Diabetes Mellitus*, London: Croom Helm.

Kantrow, A. (1963) 'A vocational and counselling service for diabetics', *Diabetes* 12 (5): 454–7.

Keen, H. (1983) 'Criteria and classification of diabetes mellitus', in J. Mann, K. Pyorala, and A. Teuscher, (eds) *Diabetes in Epidemiological Perspective*, London: Churchill Livingstone.

Keen, H. (1987) 'The genetics of diabetes: from nightmare to headache', *British Medical Journal* 294 (6577): 917–18.

Keen, H. and Ekoe, J. (1984) 'The geography of diabetes mellitus', *British Medical Journal* 40 (4): 359–65.

Keen, H., Thomas, B., Jarrett, R., and Fuller, J. (1978) 'Nutritional factors in diabetes mellitus', in J. Yudkin (ed.) *Diet of Man: Needs and Wants*, Barking, England: Applied Science Publishers.

Kelleher, D. (forthcoming) 'Coming to terms with diabetes: coping strategies and non-compliance', in R. Anderson and M. R. Bury (eds) *Living with Chronic Illness: the Experience of Patients and their Families*, Hemel Hempstead: Unwin Hyman.

Koski, M. and Kumento, A. (1977) 'The interrelationship between diabetic control and family life', *Paediatric Adolescent Endocrinology* 3: 41–5.

Lancet (1982) 'Diabetes mellitus and socio-economic factors, (editorial) 2: 530–1.

Lebovitz, H. (1985) 'Oral hypoglycaemic agents', in K. Alberti and L. Krall (eds) *The Diabetes Annual 1*, Amsterdam: Elsevier Science Publications.

Leslie, R. and Pyke, D. (1985) 'Genetics of diabetes', in K. Alberti and L. Krall (eds) *The Diabetes Annual 1*, Amsterdam: Elsevier Science Publications.

Ley, P. (1982) 'Satisfaction, compliance and communication', *British Journal of Clinical Psychology* 21: 241–54.

Lieberman, M. (1986) 'Social, supports – the consequences of psychologizing: a commentary, *Journal of Consulting and Clinical Psychology* 54 (4): 461–5.

Lindsay, M. (1985) 'Emotional management', in J. Baum and A.-L. Kinmonth (eds) *Care of the Child with Diabetes*, London: Churchill Livingstone.

Lipson, L. (1986) 'Diabetes in the elderly: diagnosis, pathogenesis, and therapy', *American Journal of Medicine* 80: 10–21.

McLean, T. (1985) *Metal Jam*, London: Hodder & Stoughton.

Malins, J. (1968) *Clinical Diabetes Mellitus*, London: Eyre & Spottiswoode.

Mason, C. (1985) 'The production and effects of uncertainty with special reference to diabetes mellitus', *Social Science and Medicine* 21 (12): 1329–34.

Mellor, J., Samanta, A., Blandford, R., and Burden, A. (1985)

'Questionnaire survey of diabetic care in general practice in Leicestershire', *Health Trends* 17: 61–3.

Minuchin, S., Rosman, B., and Baker, L. (1978) *Psychosomatic Families*, New York: Harvard University Press.

Mohan, V., Ramachandran, A. and Viswanathan, M. (1985) 'Tropical diabetes', in K. Alberti and L. Krall (eds) *The Diabetes Annual 1*, Amsterdam: Elsevier Science Publications.

Murawski, B., Chazab, B., Balodimos, M., and Ryan, J. (1970) 'Personality patterns in patients with diabetes mellitus of long duration', *Diabetes* 19: 259–63.

Nagy, V. and Wolfe, G. (1984) 'Cognitive predictors of compliance in chronic disease patients', *Medical Care* 22 (10): 912–21.

National Kidney Research Fund Report (1987) *Diabetes Mellitus and Renal Disease*, London: National Kidney Research Fund.

Nuttall, F. (1983) 'Diet and the diabetic patient', *Diabetes Care* 6 (2): 197–207.

Petrides, P. (1981) 'Sozialmedizinische problem von diabetikern, *Internist* (Berlin) 22: 242–6.

Pickup, J., Sherwin, R., Tamborlane, W., Rizza, R., and Service, F. (1985) 'The pump life: patient responses and clinical and technological problems', *Diabetes* 34 (suppl. 3).

Pollans, C. and Turkat, I. (1984) 'Effects of an insulin infusion pump and the label 'diabetes' on observers' judgements of an individual's personality and social characteristics', *Journal of Social Psychology* 19a (122): 93–9.

Porter, A. (1979) 'The Kirkcaldy Community Care Project' (unpublished report), Department of General Practice, Edinburgh University.

Revenson, T. (1983) 'Stressful life-events, coping and illness course among middle-aged and elderly diabetics', *Dissertation Abstracts International* 1 pt 43 (7–B): 2,393B.

Richards, H. (1983) 'Diabetic after-care: a study', *Balance* 21 December, London: British Diabetic Association.

Robinson, N. (1987) personal communication.

Rotter, J. (1966) 'Generalized expectancies of internal versus external control of reinforcement', *Psychological Monographs: General and Applied* 80 (1): 1–28.

Royal College of Physicians (1984) *Provision of Medical Care for Adult Diabetics in the UK*, London: Royal College of Physicians and British Diabetic Association.

Sackett, D. and Haynes, R. B. (1976) *Compliance with Therapeutic Regimens*, Baltimore, Md: Johns Hopkins University Press.

Schade, D. and Eaton, R. (1985) 'Implanted devices and the artificial pancreas', in K. Alberti and L. Krall (eds) *The Diabetes Annual 1*, Amsterdam: Elsevier Science Publications.

Schafer, L., Glasgow, R., McCaul, K., and Dreher, M. (1983) 'Adherence to IDDM regimens: relationship to psychosocial variables and metabolic control', *Diabetes Care* 6 (5): 493–8.

Schlenk, E. and Hart, L. (1984) 'Relationship between health locus of control, health value, and social support and compliance of persons with diabetes mellitus', *Diabetes Care* 7: 566–74.

Schöffling, K. Federlin, K. Ditschuneit, H., and Pfeiffer, E. (1963) 'Disorders of sexual function in male diabetics', *Diabetes* 12 (6): 519–27.

Siperstein, M., Foster, D., Knowles, H., Levine, R., Madison, L., and Roth, J. (1977) 'Control of blood glucose and diabetic vascular disease', *New England Journal of Medicine* 296 (18): 1,060–2.

Sonksen, P., Ryle A., and Milton, J. (1987) 'Poor diabetic control resulting from psychological factors: the efficacy of brief psychotherapy' (personal communication).

Spencer, K. and Cudworth, A. (1983) 'The aetiology of insulin-dependent diabetes mellitus' in J. Mann, K. Pyorala, and A. Teuscher (eds) *Diabetes in Epidemiological Perspective*, London: Churchill Livingstone.

Stone, D. (1961) 'A study of the incidence and causes of poor control in patients with diabetes mellitus', *American Journal of the Medical Sciences* 241: 436–41.

Strauss, A. and Glaser, B. (1975) *Chronic Illness and the Quality of Life*, St Louis MO: Mosby.

Stuart, S. (1971) 'Day to day with diabetes', *American Journal of Nursing* 71 (8): 1548–50.

Sullivan, B.-J. (1979) 'Adjustment in adolescent girls: (1) development of the diabetic adjustment scale', *Psychosomatic Medicine* 41 (2): 119–26.

Surwit, R., Scovern, A., and Feinglos, M. (1982) 'The role of behaviour in diabetes care', *Diabetes Care* 5 (3): 337–42.

Sutherland, D., Kendall, D., Goetz, F., and Najarian, J. (1985) 'Pancreas transplantation in man', in K. Alberti and L. Krall (eds) *The Diabetes Annual 1*, Amsterdam: Elsevier Science Publications.

Tasker, P. (1986) 'Your GP and you', *Balance* Dec/Jan. London: British Diabetic Association.

Tattersall, R. (1985) 'Self-monitoring of blood glucose 1978–1984', in K. Alberti and L. Krall (eds) *The Diabetes Annual 1*, Amsterdam: Elsevier Science Publications.

Tattersall, R. and Jackson, J. (1982) 'Social and emotional complications of diabetes', in R. Jarrett and H. Keen (eds) *Complications of Diabetes* (2nd edn) London: Arnold.

Tattersall, R. and Walford, S. (1985) 'Brittle diabetes in response to life-stress: cheating and manipulation', in J. Pickup (ed.) *Brittle Diabetes*, Oxford: Blackwell Scientific Publications.

Taylor, R. and Zimmet, P. (1983) 'Migrant studies in diabetes epidemiology', in J. Mann, K. Pyorala, and A. Teuscher, (eds) *Diabetes in Epidemiological Perspective*, London: Churchill Livingstone.

Thomas, B. (1981) 'How successful are we at persuading diabetics to follow their diet – and why do we sometimes fail?' in M. Turner and B. Thomas (eds) *Nutrition and Diabetes*, London: J. Libbey.

Thorn, P. A. (1974) 'On looking after diabetic patients – hospital clinic or practice mini-clinic', *Midland Medical Review* 7: 151–4.

Treuting, T. (1961) 'The role of emotional factors in the etiology and course of diabetes mellitus: a review of the recent literature', *American Journal of the Medical Sciences* 244: 131–47.

Tunbridge, R. and Weatherill, J. (1970) 'Reliability and cost of diabetic diets', *British Medical Journal* 2: 78–80.

Wallston, K., Wallston, B., and DeVellis, R. (1978) 'Development of multi-dimensional health locus of control (MHLC) scales', *Health Education Monographs* 6.

Walsh, C. (1983) 'Menstruation and Diabetes', *Balance* August: 11, London: British Diabetic Association.

Ward, J. (1985) 'Diabetic neuropathy', in K. Alberti and L. Krall (eds) *The Diabetes Annual 1*, Amsterdam: Elsevier Science Publications.

Ward, J. (1986) 'Guidelines for using insulin infusion pumps', *Diabetes Update* 9 (August), London: British Diabetic Association.

Watkin, J., Williams, F., Martin, D., Hogan, M., and Anderson, E. (1967) 'A study of diabetic patients at home', *American Journal of Public Health* 57: 452–9.

Watkins, P. (1984) 'Pain and diabetic neuropathy', *British Medical Journal* 21 January: 168–9.

Weiner, C. (1975) 'The burden of rheumatoid arthritis: tolerating the uncertainty', *Social Science and Medicine* 9: 97–104.

West, K. M. (1973) 'Diet therapy of diabetes: an analysis of failure', *Annals of Internal Medicine* 79: 425–34.

West, K. M. (1982) 'Hyperglycaemia as a cause of long-term complications', in H. Keen and R. J. Jarrett (eds) *Complications of Diabetes* (2nd edn) London: Arnold.

WHO (1985) *Diabetes Mellitus Technical Report Series 727*, Geneva: World Health Organisation.

Wierenga, M. (1984) 'The interrelationship between multi-dimensional health locus of control, knowledge of diabetes, perceived social support, self-reported compliance and therapeutic outcomes 6 weeks after the adult patient has been diagnosed with DM, *Dissertation Abstracts International* 40: 5,610B.

Williams, H. (1985) 'Diabetes in general practice', *Diabetes Update* November: 1–3, London: British Diabetic Association.

Yudkin, J., Boucher, B., and Schopfein, K. (1980) 'The quality of diabetic care in a London health district', *Journal of Epidemiology and Community Health* 34: 277–80.

Zimmet, P. (1982) 'Type 2 (non-insulin – dependent) diabetes – an epidemiological overview', *Diabetologia* 22: 399–411.

Name index

Subject index